HEALTH:
OUR GREATEST WEALTH
a health and wellness guide

HEALTH:
OUR GREATEST WEALTH

a health and wellness guide

Bonnie Labuda and Mary Mueller

BALBOA.
PRESS
A DIVISION OF HAY HOUSE

ISBN: 978-1-4525-5334-4 (sc)
ISBN: 978-1-4525-5335-1 (e)
ISBN: 978-1-4525-5336-8 (hc)

Library of Congress Control Number: 2012909862

Balboa Press books may be ordered through booksellers or by contacting:

Balboa Press
A Division of Hay House
1663 Liberty Drive
Bloomington, IN 47403
www.balboapress.com
1-(877) 407-4847

Because of the dynamic nature of the Internet, any web addresses or links contained in this book may have changed since publication and may no longer be valid. The views expressed in this work are solely those of the author and do not necessarily reflect the views of the publisher, and the publisher hereby disclaims any responsibility for them.

The author of this book does not dispense medical advice or prescribe the use of any technique as a form of treatment for physical, emotional, or medical problems without the advice of a physician, either directly or indirectly. The intent of the author is only to offer information of a general nature to help you in your quest for emotional and spiritual well-being. In the event you use any of the information in this book for yourself, which is your constitutional right, the author and the publisher assume no responsibility for your actions.

Any people depicted in stock imagery provided by Thinkstock are models, and such images are being used for illustrative purposes only.
Certain stock imagery © Thinkstock.

Printed in the United States of America

Balboa Press rev. date: 08/28/2012

About the Authors

Hello!, I'm Bonnie LaBuda, owner and founder of Herb n' Essences. I grew up on a 160-acre hobby farm south of St. Cloud, Minnesota. I spent a lot of my childhood with my grandmother, Laurie, who was a wonderful woman. At the time, she hadn't realized she was both a nutritionist and an herbalist! From her, I learned a great deal about nutrition and herbs, knowledge that, I treasure today, as an adult.

In the early '90s, I studied the alternative therapies of acupressure, massage, and aromatherapy. For one summer in the mid-1990s, I studied with an herbalist. Herbalism, I learned, is definitely a calling! In 2000, I started working with an herbalist and biochemist. Together, we developed the products I now sell at my website, herbnessences.com. I am so appreciative and thankful to God for all the wonderful gifts He has put on this earth for our use and good health.

If you have questions, please feel free to contact me at (320) 252-5745.

Hello! I'm Mary Mueller.

I'm an avid gardener. My garden contains literally hundreds of perennials, and I've dedicated a sizeable portion of my garden space to vegetables and herbs. Throughout the winter, my family enjoys the fruits of our labor with frozen and canned fruits and vegetables. Because we eat truly 'local' foods, my husband and I are eating better, more healthfully. Growing our own food is a blessing in and of itself!

For more than 16 years, I have also worked in the technology field. My expertise lies in web design, content, and user experience, as well as in training and productivity. I have also worked in support and design. I enjoy helping people use technology to spread their message.

I invite you to visit my website, www.techlenz.com.

Dedications

Bonnie's:

To my son Cole, who has been my greatest teacher, inspiring me to always reach higher.

Love Mom

Mary's:

To my husband Greg, who supports all of my wishes and dreams.

Contents

FOODS

ACID/ALKALINE FOODS

HEALTHY TIP #1: Throughout the day, sip ice water.

Eight 16 oz glasses per day helps hydrate cells and burn calories

(Approximately 200 calories per day)

BALANCING THE BODY'S PH IS A MAJOR PART OF WELL-BEING AND GREATER HEALTH.

pH scale: 0 1 2 3 4 5 6 7 healthy 8 9 10 11 12 13 14

(Bonnie) Well, I can honestly say that when I'm eating a healthy diet with a good P.H., I feel better, have more energy and am more creative, and sleep better.

I've had several acquaintances over the years that have used just the P.H. diet alone to cure cancer.

What the numbers mean: A pH of 7.0 is neutral. A pH below 7.0 is acidic. A pH above 7.0 is alkaline. Above or below the desired range brings on symptoms of disease, or disease itself. Human blood pH should be slightly alkaline (7.35 to 7.45).

Eating acid-forming diets, emotional stress, toxic overload, and/or immune reactions, or any process that deprives the cells of oxygen and other nutrients are all things that may create an acidic pH. To compensate, the body uses available stores of alkaline minerals. What happens if there are not enough minerals to overcome that loss? Acids build up in our cells. An acidic balance decreases

- o the body's ability to absorb minerals and other nutrients;
- o decrease energy production in cells;
- o decrease the body's ability to repair damaged cells;
- o decrease its ability to detoxify heavy metals.

An acidic balance may cause tumor cells to thrive, and it can make the body more susceptible to fatigue and illness. A blood pH of 6.9, which is only slightly acidic, can induce coma and death.

Acidosis has become more common in our society, mostly due to the typical American diet: far too high in acid-producing animal products like meat, eggs, and dairy, and far too low in alkaline-producing foods like fresh vegetables. Processed foods, such as white flour and sugar, produce acids, as do coffee and soft drinks. We also use too many drugs, another acid-forming source. And we use artificial chemical sweeteners, such as NutraSweet, Spoonful, Sweet 'N Low, Equal, or Aspartame, all poisonous and extremely acid-forming. Cleaning up our diets and our lifestyles are two of the best habits we can develop to correct overly-acidic bodies. Strive for these percentages:

60/40: To maintain health, the diet should consist of 60% alkaline-forming foods and 40% acid-forming foods.

80/20: To restore health, the diet should consist of 80% alkaline-forming foods and 20% acid-forming foods.

Generally, alkaline-forming foods include most fruits, green vegetables, peas, beans, lentils, spices, herbs and seasonings, seeds, and nuts.

Generally, acid-forming foods include meat, fish, poultry, eggs, grains, and legumes.

Shifting Your pH Towards Alkaline

To adjust your body's pH, use the following food lists as a general guide to alkaline and acidic foods. Always remember that an acidic body is a sickness magnet. What you eat and drink will impact where your body's pH level falls. Balance is **key** !!!

Source: Rense, James. *Rense.com*. A list of Acid / Alkaline Forming Foods. <http://www.rense.com/1.mpicons/acidalka.htm>

ALKALINE FOODS

Vegetables - Alfalfa, Barley Grass, Beet Greens, Beets, Broccoli, Cabbage, Carrots, Cauliflower, Celery, Chard, Greens, Chlorella, Collard Greens, Cucumbers, Dandelions, Dulce, Edible Flowers, Eggplant, Fermented Veggies, Garlic, Green Beans, Green Peas, Kale, Kohlrabi, Lettuce, Mushrooms, Mustard Greens, Nightshade Veggies, Onions, Parsnips (High Glycemic), Peas, Peppers, Pumpkin, Radishes, Rutabaga, Sea Veggies, Spinach Greens, Spirulina, Sprouts, Sweet Potatoes, Tomatoes, Watercress, Wheat Grass, Wild Greens.

Oriental Vegetables – Daikon, Dandelion Root, Kombu, Maitake, Nori, Reishi, Shitake, Umeboshi, Wakame.

Fruits - Apples, Apricots, Avocadoes, Bananas (High Glycemic), Berries, Blackberries, Cantaloupe, Cherries (Sour), Coconut (Fresh), Currants, Dates (Dried), Figs (Dried), Grapes, Grapefruit, Honeydew Melon, Lemons, Limes, Muskmelons, Nectarines, Oranges, Peaches, Pears, Pineapple, Raisins, Raspberries, Rhubarb, Strawberries, Tangerines, Tomatoes, Tropical Fruits, Umeboshi Plums, Watermelon.

Proteins - Almonds, Chestnuts, Millet, Tempeh (Fermented), Tofu (Fermented), Whey Protein Powder.

Sweeteners – Stevia.

Spices and Seasonings - Chili Peppers, Cinnamon, Curry, Ginger, Herbs (All), Miso, Mustard, Sea Salt, Tamari

Other - Alkaline Antioxidant Water, Apple Cider Vinegar, Bee Pollen, Fresh Fruit Juice, Green Juices, Lecithin Granules, Mineral Water, Molasses, Blackstrap, Probiotic Cultures, Soured Dairy Products, Veggie Juices.

Minerals - Calcium: pH 12, Cesium: pH 14, Magnesium: pH 9, Potassium: pH 14, Sodium: pH 14.

ACIDIC FOODS

Vegetables – Corn, Lentils, Olives, Winter Squash.

Fruits – Blueberries, Canned or Glazed Fruits, Cranberries, Currants, Plums**, Prunes**.

Grains, Grain Products – Amaranth, Barley, Bran (Oat), Bran (Wheat), Bread, Corn, Cornstarch, Crackers (Soda), Flour (Wheat), Flour (White), Hemp Seed Flour, Kamut, Macaroni, Noodles, Oatmeal, Oats (Rolled), Quinoa, Rice (All), Rice Cakes, Rye, Spaghetti, Spelt, Wheat Germ, Wheat.

Beans & Legumes - Black Beans, Chick Peas, Green Peas, Kidney Beans, Lentils, Pinto Beans, Red Beans, Soy Beans, White Beans

Dairy – Butter, Cheese, Cheese (Processed), Ice Cream, Ice Milk.

Nuts & Butters – Cashews, Legumes, Peanut Butter, Peanuts, Pecans, Tahini, Walnuts.

Animal Protein – Bacon, Beef, Carp, Clams, Cod, Corned Beef, Fish, Haddock, Lamb, Lobster, Mussels, Organ Meats, Oyster, Pike, Pork, Rabbit, Salmon, Sardines, Sausage, Scallops, Shellfish, Shrimp, Tuna, Turkey, Veal, Venison.

Fats & Oils - Avocado Oil, Butter, Canola Oil, Corn Oil, Flax Oil, Hemp Seed Oil, Lard, Olive Oil, Safflower Oil, Sesame Oil, Sunflower Oil.

Sweeteners – Carob, Corn Syrup, Sugar.

Alcohol – Beer, Hard Liquor, Spirits, Wine.

Other Foods – Catsup, Cocoa, Coffee, Mustard, Pepper, Soft Drinks, Vinegar (White).

Drugs & Chemicals – Aspirin, Chemicals, Drugs (Medicinal), Drugs (Psychedelic), Herbicides, Pesticides, Tobacco.

Junk Food - Beer: pH 2.5, Coca-Cola: pH 2, Coffee: pH 4.

FOODS RANKED ALKALINE TO ACIDIC

Extremely Alkaline - Lemons, watermelon.

Alkaline-Forming - Cantaloupe, Cayenne, Celery, Dates, Figs, Kelp, Limes, Mango, Melons, Papaya, Parsley, Seaweeds, Seedless Grapes (Sweet), Watercress. Asparagus, Fruit Juices, Grapes (Sweet), Kiwifruit, Passion Fruit, Pears (Sweet), Pineapple, Raisins, Umeboshi Plums, and Vegetable Juices.

Moderately Alkaline - Apples (Sweet), Alfalfa Sprouts, Apricots, Avocadoes, Bananas (Ripe), Currants, Dates, Figs (Fresh), Garlic, Grapefruit, Grapes (Less Sweet), Guavas, Herbs (Leafy Green), Lettuce (Leafy Green), Nectarine, Peaches (Sweet), Pears (Less Sweet), Peas (Fresh, Sweet), Pumpkin (Sweet), Sea Salt (Vegetable).

Apples (Sour), Beans (Fresh, Green), Beets, Bell Peppers, Broccoli, Cabbage, Carob, Cauliflower, Ginger (Fresh), Grapes (Sour), Lettuce (Pale Green), Oranges, Peaches (Less Sweet), Peas (Less Sweet), Potatoes (With Skin), Pumpkin (Less Sweet), Raspberries, Strawberries, Squash, Sweet Corn (Fresh), Turnips, Vinegar (Apple Cider).

Slightly Alkaline - Almonds, artichokes (Jerusalem), Brussels Sprouts, Cherries, Coconut (Fresh), Cucumbers, Eggplant, Honey (Raw), Leeks, Mushrooms, Okra, Olives (Ripe), Onions, Pickles (Homemade), Radishes, Sea Salt, Spices, Tomatoes (Sweet), Vinegar (Sweet Brown Rice).

Chestnuts (Dry, Roasted), Egg Yolks (Soft Cooked), Essene Bread, Goat's Milk and Whey (Raw), Mayonnaise (Homemade), Olive Oil, Sesame Seeds (Whole), Soybeans (Dry), Soy Cheese, Soy Milk, Sprouted Grains, Tofu, Tomatoes (Less Sweet), and Yeast (Nutritional Flakes).

Neutral - Butter (Fresh, Unsalted), Cream (Fresh, Raw), Cow's Milk and Whey (Raw), Margarine, Oils (Except Olive), and Yogurt (Plain).

Moderately Acidic - Bananas (Green), Barley (Rye), Blueberries, Bran, Butter, Cereals (Unrefined), Cheeses, Crackers (Unrefined Rye,

Rice, and Wheat), Cranberries, Dried Beans (Mung, Adzuki, Pinto, Kidney, Garbanzo), Dry Coconut, Egg Whites, Eggs Whole (Cooked Hard), Fructose, Goat's Milk (Homogenized), Honey (Pasteurized), Ketchup, Maple Syrup (Unprocessed), Milk (Homogenized).

Molasses (Unsulfured and Organic), Most Nuts, Mustard, Oats (Rye, Organic), Olives (Pickled), Pasta (Whole Grain), Pastry (Whole Grain and Honey), Plums, Popcorn (With Salt and/or Butter), Potatoes, Prunes, Rice (Basmati and Brown), Seeds (Pumpkin, Sunflower), Soy Sauce, and Wheat Bread (Sprouted Organic).

Extremely Acidic - Artificial Sweeteners, Beef, Beer, Breads, Brown Sugar, Carbonated Soft Drinks, Cereals (Refined), Chocolate, Cigarettes and Tobacco, Coffee, Cream of Wheat (Unrefined), Custard (With White Sugar), Deer, Drugs, Fish, Flour (White, Wheat), Fruit Juices with Sugar, Jams, Jellies, Lamb.

Liquor, Maple Syrup (Processed), Molasses (Sulfured), Pasta (White), Pastries and Cakes from White Flour, Pickles (Commercial), Pork, Poultry, Seafood, Sugar (White), Table Salt (Refined and Iodized), Tea (Black), White Bread, White Vinegar (Processed), Whole Wheat Foods, Wine, and Yogurt (Sweetened).

Highly Alkaline-Forming Foods - Baking Soda, Sea Salt, Mineral Water, Pumpkin Seeds, Lentils, Seaweed, Onions, Taro Root, Sea Vegetables, Lotus Root, Sweet Potatoes, Limes, Lemons, Nectarines, Persimmons, Raspberries, Watermelon, Tangerines, and Pineapple

Moderately Alkaline-Forming Foods - Apricots, Spices, Kombucha, Unsulfured Molasses, Soy Sauce, Cashews, Chestnuts, Pepper, Kohlrabi, Parsnips, Garlic, Asparagus, Kale, Parsley, Endive, Arugula, Mustard Green, Ginger Root, Broccoli, Grapefruit, Cantaloupe, Honeydew, Citrus, Olives, Dewberry, Carrots, Loganberry, and Mango.

Low Alkaline-Forming Foods - Most herbs, Green Tea, Mu Tea, Rice Syrup, Apple Cider Vinegar, Sake, Quail Eggs, Primrose Oil, Sesame Seeds, Cod Liver Oil, Almonds, Sprouts, Potatoes (White), Bell Pepper, Mushrooms, Cauliflower, Cabbage, Rutabaga, Ginseng, Eggplant, Pumpkin, Collard Green, Pears, Avocadoes, Apples (Sour), Blackberries, Cherries, Peaches, and Papaya.

Very Low Alkaline-Forming Foods - Ginger Tea, Umeboshi Vinegar, Ghee, Duck Eggs, Oats, Grain Coffee, Quinoa, Japonica Rice, Wild Rice, Avocado Oil, Most Seeds, Coconut Oil, Olive Oil, Flax Oil, Brussels Sprouts, Beets, Chive, Cilantro, Celery, Okra, Cucumbers, Turnip Greens, Squashes, Lettuces, Oranges, Bananas, Blueberries, Raisins, Currants, Grapes, and Strawberries.

Very Low Acid-Forming Foods - Curry, Kona Coffee, Honey, Maple Syrup, Vinegar, Cream, Butter, Goat/Sheep Cheese, Chicken, Gelatin, Organs, Venison, Fish, Wild Duck, Triticale, Millet, Kashi, Amaranth, Brown Rice, Pumpkin Seed Oil, Grape Seed Oil, Sunflower Oil, Pine Nuts, Canola Oil, Spinach, Fava Beans, Black-Eyed Peas, String Beans, Wax Beans, Zucchini, Chutney, Rhubarb, Coconut, Guava, Dry Fruit, Figs, and Dates.

Low Acid-Forming Foods - Vanilla, Alcohol, Black Tea, Balsamic Vinegar, Cow's Milk, Aged Cheese, Soy Cheese, Goat's Milk, Game Meat, Lamb, Mutton, Boar, Elk, Shellfish, Mollusks, Goose, Turkey, Buckwheat, Wheat, Spelt, Teff, Kamut, Farina, Semolina, White Rice, Almond Oil, Sesame Oil, Safflower Oil, Tapioca, Seitan, Tofu, Pinto Beans, White Beans, Navy Beans, Red Beans, Adzuki Beans, Lima Beans, Chard, Plums, Prunes, and Tomatoes.

Moderately Acid-Forming Foods - Nutmeg, Coffee, Casein, Milk Protein, Cottage Cheese, Pork, Veal, Bear, Mussels, Squid, Chicken, Maize, Barley Groats, Corn, Rye, Oat Bran, Pistachio Seeds, Chestnut Oil, Lard, Pecans, Palm Kernel Oil, Green Peas, Peanuts, Snow Peas, Other Legumes, Garbanzo Beans, Cranberries, and Pomegranate.

Highly Acid-Forming Foods - Tabletop Sweeteners (NutraSweet, Spoonful, Sweet 'N Low, Equal, or Aspartame), Pudding, Jam, Jelly, Table Salt (NaCl), Beer, Yeast, Hops, Malt, Sugar, Cocoa, White (Acetic Acid) Vinegar, Processed Cheese, Ice Cream, Beef, Lobster, Pheasant, Barley, Cottonseed Oil, Hazelnuts, Walnuts, Brazil Nuts, Fried Foods, Soybeans, and Soft Drinks (especially Colas. To neutralize a glass of cola with a pH of 2.5, it would take 32 glasses of alkaline water with a pH of 10.)

This chart is ©2012 Essense-of-Life, LLC. Used with permission.

Source: <http://www.essense-of-life.com/moreinfo/healthtopics/A-701/
foodcharts.htm>

HEALTHY TIP #2: Minimize noise in your life.

Spend more time outdoors listening to nature sounds.

**Every day, for 5 to 10 minutes, lie down, inside
or outside, listening to nature sounds.**

HONEY and CINNAMON

THEIR BENEFITS

HEALTHY TIP #3: Spend time in the sun.

Each day, spend 10 minutes in the sun without sunscreen or sunglasses (before 10:00 a.m. or after 3:00 p.m.)

Indoors, replace incandescent or fluorescent bulbs with full-spectrum bulbs.

(Bonnie) In many books and on the Internet, the benefits of honey and cinnamon are touted. I have used all of these remedies with clients for years. They are amazed at the healing power of these remedies.

Personally, my son had pneumonia at age 7; he was on antibiotics for four weeks with no relief. The doctors took him off the meds and told us to come back in two weeks. I called my grandmother; she said to use honey and lemon - 1 teaspoon every hour after breakfast. In 2 days the cough was totally gone.

Honey and Cinnamon have many health benefits. Honey has been used for its medicinal purposes for many years.

It is useful in fighting heart disease, insect bites, reducing cholesterol and curing the common cold. Honey can be used without side effects. It is also sweet without harmful side effects for diabetic patients.

Strengthen Heart Muscles: Make a paste of honey and cinnamon powder, apply on bread, or other bread, instead of jelly and jam and eat it regularly for breakfast. It can reduce the cholesterol in the arteries and prevent additional heart attacks.

Regular use of the above process relieves loss of breath and strengthens the heartbeat

Bug Bites: Take one part honey to two parts of lukewarm water and add a small teaspoon of cinnamon powder, make a paste and massage it on the itching part of the body slowly. It is noticed that the pain recedes within a minute or two.

Arthritis: Arthritis patients may take daily, morning and night, one cup of hot water with two spoons of honey and one small teaspoon of cinnamon powder. If taken regularly even chronic arthritis can be cured.

Baldness: Those suffering from hair loss or baldness, may apply a paste of hot olive oil, one tablespoon of honey, one teaspoon of cinnamon powder before bath and keep it on for approx. 15 min. and then wash the hair. It was found to be effective even if kept on for 5 minutes.

Urinary Track Health: Take two tablespoons of cinnamon powder and one teaspoon of honey in a glass of lukewarm water and drink it. It destroys the germs in the bladder.

Toothache: Make a paste of one teaspoon of cinnamon powder and five teaspoons of honey and apply on the aching tooth. This may be applied 3 times a day till the tooth stops aching.

Cholesterol: Two tablespoons of honey and three teaspoons of Cinnamon Powder mixed in 16 ounces of tea water, given to a cholesterol patient, was found to reduce the level of cholesterol in the blood by 10% within 2 hours. As mentioned for arthritic patients, if taken 3 times a day, any Chronic cholesterol is cured. As per information received in the said journal, pure honey taken with food daily relieves complaints of cholesterol.

Colds: Those suffering from common or severe colds should take one tablespoon lukewarm honey with 1/4 spoon cinnamon powder daily for 3 days. This process will cure most chronic cough, cold and clear the sinuses.

Strengthen Immune System: Daily use of honey and cinnamon powder strengthens the immune system and protects the body from bacteria and viral attacks. Scientists have found that honey has various vitamins and iron in large amounts. Constant use of honey strengthens the white blood corpuscles to fight bacteria and viral diseases.

Upset Stomach: Cinnamon powder sprinkled on two tablespoons of honey taken before food, relieves acidity and digests the heaviest of meals. Honey taken with cinnamon powder cures stomachache and also clears stomach ulcers from the root.

Flu: A scientist in Spain has proved that honey contains a natural ingredient, which kills the influenza germs and saves the patient from flu.

Vitality as a person ages: Tea made with honey and cinnamon powder, when taken regularly arrests the ravages of old age. Take 4 spoons of honey, 1 spoon of cinnamon powder and 3 cups of water and boil to make like tea. Drink 1/4 cup, 3 to 4 times a day. It keeps the skin fresh and soft and arrests old age.

Clear Skin: Three tablespoons of Honey and one teaspoon of cinnamon powder paste. Apply this paste on the pimples before sleeping and wash it the next morning with warm water. If done daily for two weeks, it removes pimples from the root.

Skin Afflictions: Applying honey and cinnamon powder in equal parts on the affected parts cures eczema, ringworm and all types of skin infections.

Weight Control: Daily in the morning 1/2 hour before breakfast on an empty stomach and at night before sleeping, drink honey and cinnamon powder boiled in one-cup water. If taken regularly it reduces the weight of even the most obese person.

Also, drinking of this mixture regularly does not allow the fat to accumulate in the body even though the person may eat a high calorie diet.

Cancer prevention: Recent research in Japan and Australia has revealed that advanced cancer of the stomach and bones have been cured successfully. Patients suffering from these kinds of cancer should daily take one tablespoon of honey with one teaspoon of cinnamon powder for one month 3 times a day.

Tiredness: Recent studies have shown that the sugar content of honey is more helpful rather than being detrimental to the strength of the body. Senior citizens, who take honey and cinnamon powder in equal parts, are more alert and flexible.

Bad Breath: Gargle in the morning with one teaspoon of honey and cinnamon powder mixed in hot water. Your breath will stay fresh throughout the day.

Improve Hearing: Daily morning and night honey and cinnamon powder taken in equal parts restore hearing.

(Mary) As a child growing up, when I had a sore throat, my mother would heat up water and add honey to the heated water. This was an instant help and would help soothe the pain.

HEALTHY TIP #4: Spend time with pets, or with neighbors or friends' pets.

Animals love unconditionally and change our mood

COLLECTING HERBS

HEALTHY TIP #5: Spend time with children (those you really like!).

(Bonnie) My whole life, spring has always been my favorite time of the year.

As a child, I was fascinated by spring time, everything was popping out of the ground, I knew in my little soul it all had a purpose.

To take my first herb classes years ago was wonderful. We got to learn about barks, herbs, roots – it was a dream come true to learn why God had put it all here.

Gather herbs from early spring through late autumn. Collect them on sunny days, for the potency is considerably higher then. Pick herbs far away from polluted areas like roadside ditches, cities, industrial areas. Make sure the herbs have not been treated with fertilizers or pesticides.

Bark: Collect in early spring, before the trees bud.

Leaves: Collect before they turn to seed or fruit.

Roots: Collect in the fall after leaves have fallen from the plant.

Plants: Cut off at least 2 inches above ground. Never pull plants out by the roots. Always leave some of the plant so that it reseeds in that area. Thank your plants and leave a gift such as tobacco in the area where you harvested. Respect and Gratitude are very important.

Storing and Drying Herbs

Place finely-chopped roots, leaves, barks on a clean cloth or sheet, and lay them out to dry in an airy, shady spot. Do not wash unless drying roots. (If drying them, use only clean, unpolluted water.) Once herbs are dried, store in a cardboard box, brown paper bag, or in dark glass jars. Store away from sunlight.

How to Prepare Herbs

Capsule: Taking herbs in capsules is easy, convenient, and you avoid the bitter taste, a method most people prefer. Capsules also save on preparation, while providing an exact, regulated dosage to the body.

Decoction: Simmer herbs, usually one part plant to twenty parts water, uncovered, for 10 to 20 minutes until one-third of the water has decreased through evaporation. Decoction extracts the deeper essences from harder or coarser herbs, such as stems, barks, and roots. Note: For coarser herbs, such as Valerian and Burdock, simmer gently in a covered pot to bring out their medicinal properties. Strain before using.

Tinctures: Fill a glass jar with fresh-picked or dried herbs. Cover completely with 60 proof, or higher, alcohol. (You may prefer flavored vodka or brandy.) Seal the jar and keep out of sunlight. Shake twice daily for two weeks; strain, using cheesecloth. Store in a dark glass bottle.

Oils: Tightly press herbs into a bowl. Cover with cold-pressed olive oil. Place in oven at 225 degrees for 2-1/2 hours. Cool; strain and place in dark glass bottles. Exact dosages are recommended on individual bottles. Check with local herbalist on dosages. Always mark the date, and location where you picked the herbs, on the bottle.

Fomentation: To prepare a fomentation, soak a towel or cloth in the desired tea, as hot as can be tolerated without burning, then apply the towel to the affected area. Cover the towel with a dry flannel cloth. Repeat, as needed. A fomentations is an external application of herbs, generally used to treat swelling, pain, cold, and flu.

Infusion: Pour a cup of boiling water over a teaspoon (the usual amount) of leaves, blossoms, or flowers. Steep for three to five minutes; strain before drinking. Add honey, if desired. Infusions extract an herb's active properties by steeping or soaking, usually in water. It's the common way to prepare herbs.

Plaster: A plaster is much like a poultice. It prevents irritation to the skin by placing herbal materials between two pieces of cloth before applying to the affected area.

Poultice: To prepare a poultice, add enough hot water to make a thick paste. Apply directly to the skin. Cover with a hot, moist towel. Leave on until the paste cools. Repeat, as needed. A poultice acts as an antiseptic to reduce swelling by applying a warm mass of powdered herbs directly to the skin.

Salve: Follow procedure, as for oil. Place oil in glass measuring bowl. Heat on low. Add 1/4 teaspoon of beeswax for each cup of oil. When beeswax has melted, cool and pour into jars. More or less beeswax can be used to reach desired consistency.

Vitamins, Minerals, Trace Minerals, and Their Herb Sources

Many herbs are excellent for ingesting to provide the body with the vitamins and minerals it needs. The body usually digests them easier through plants than through fish or animal sources. Below are vitamins, minerals, and trace minerals, and their herb sources:

Vitamin A: Alfalfa, Cayenne, Eyebright, Lambs Quarter, Paprika, Red Clover, Violet, Yellow Dock

Vitamin B: Alfalfa, Dulse, Fenugreek, Kelp, Licorice, Saffron

Vitamin C: Bee Pollen, Chickweed, Echinacea,, Garlic, Goldenseal, Juniper Berries, Paprika, Peppermint, Rosehips, Sorrell, Violet, Watercress

Vitamin D: Alfalfa, Dandelion, Red Raspberry, Rosehips, Sarsaparilla, Watercress

Vitamin E: Alfalfa, Burdock, Dandelion, Dong Quai, Kelp, Scullcap, Sesame, Slippery Elm, Watercress

Vitamin G: Fo-ti-tieng

Vitamin K: Alfalfa, Gotu Kola, Shepherd's Purse

Niacin: Alfalfa, Fenugreek, Parsley, Watercress

Vitamin P: Rutin, Bioflavenoids, Acerola, Paprika

MINERALS

Calcium: Aloe, Cayenne, Chamomile, Fennel, Marshmallow, Sage, White Oak Bark

Cobalt: Dandelion, Horsetail, Juniper Berries, Lobelia, Parsley, Red Clover, White Oak Bark

Iodine: Bladderwack, Kelp

Iron: Burdock, Chickweed, Ginseng, Hops, Mullein, Nettles, Peppermint, Rosemary, Sarsaparilla, Scullcap, Yellow Dock

Magnesium: Alfalfa, Catnip, Ginger, Gotu Kola, Red Clover, Rosemary, Valerian, Wood Betony

Potassium: Aloe, Cayenne, Fennel, Goldenseal, Parsley, Rosehips, Slippery Elm, Valerian

Zinc: Burdock, Chamomile, Dandelion, Eyebright, Marshmallow, Sarsaparilla

Trace Minerals: Alfalfa, Burdock, Dandelion, Kelp, Yellow Dock, Parsley, Red Clover, Rosehips, Sage, Sarsaparilla, Valerian.

(Mary) As an avid gardener, I love planting herbs and using them fresh every day in my cooking and then using dried herbs in cooking and for improving health. Also, all of the herbs available in nature, expand my garden every day of the growing season.

HEALTHY TIP #6: Stretching and breathing a few times daily helps reduce stress and energize the body.

ORGANIC FOOD

(Bonnie) I grew up on an organic farm – we had a huge garden and canned everything in the fall. We had fruit trees; we raised our own chickens and beef. I remember Mom used to cultivate our crops and my brothers and sisters and I weeded the garden. There were never any chemicals used on our farms. I believe that genetically altering our food supply, spraying chemicals on them, giving hormones to our animals is going to have a devastating long term effect on our health and wellbeing.

Organic foods are produced utilizing environmentally-sound methods that thoroughly avoid modern synthetic inputs, such as pesticides and chemical fertilizers, irradiation, industrial solvents, or chemical food additives. Organic foods are not grown or raised utilizing any of the biotechnical industry's genetically modified organisms (GMOs).

For the majority of mankind's history, agriculture could be correctly described as "organic." Then, in the 20th Century, a great number of new synthetic chemicals were introduced into our food supply. In the 1940s, the organic farming kineticism, known as the Green Revolution, arose in replication to the industrialization of agriculture.

Origin and Meaning of the Term

IThe holistic, ecologically-balanced approach to farming greatly contrasted with what he called "chemical farming," which relied on "imported fertility" and "cannot be self-sufficient nor an organic whole." This use of "organic" differs from the scientific use of the term, which refers to a class of molecules that contain carbon, especially those involved in the chemistry of life.

Bonnie Labuda and Mary Mueller

Identifying Organic Food

According to the U.S. Organic Foods Production Act, processed organic foods usually contain only organic ingredients. If non-organic ingredients are present, at least a certain percentage---95% in the United States,[7] Canada, and Australia—of the food's total plant and animal ingredients must be organic. Foods claiming to be organic must be free of artificial food additives. They're often processed with fewer artificial methods, materials, chemical ripening, food irradiation, and genetically-modified (GMO) ingredients. An exception is made for non-synthetic pesticides. Non-organically produced ingredients are subject to various agricultural requirements.

Early consumers of organic food probed for fresh or minimally-processed foods, those utilizing only approved pesticides, those not chemically treated. Mostly, they bought directly from growers, observing this motto: "Know your farmer, know your food." By talking to farmers, observing farm conditions and farming activities, they developed their own definitions of what constituted "organic." While savvy consumers monitored them, diminutively minuscule farmers, organically certified or not, used organic farming practices to grow vegetables and raise livestock. Authoritatively mandate for organic foods incremented to new levels. Mass outlets like supermarkets reaped high-volume sales, and rapidly superseded the direct-farmer connection. Today, organic farms are not limited to size; many large corporate farms have an organic division. However, consumers of supermarket organic foods must rely on "certified organic" labeling since they are unable to facilely observe, as did early organic consumers, how their foods are grown. They look to government regulations and additional inspectors for assurance.

The USDA routinely inspects farms that produce foods bearing the USDA certified organic seal. Fifteen of the 30 third-party inspectors have been placed on probation after an auditor exposed major gaps in federal oversight of the organic food industrury. On April 20, 2010, the Department of Agriculture announced it would begin enforcing rules requiring spot-testing of organically-grown foods for traces of pesticides.

Environmental Impact

Countless surveys and studies have examined and compared conventional and organic systems of farming. The general consensus: Organic farming is less damaging for the following reasons:

- Organic farms do not consume or release synthetic pesticides into the environment. Some have the potential to harm soil, water, and local terrestrial and aquatic wildlife.

- Organic farms outperform conventional farms at sustaining diverse ecosystems, i.e., plant and insect populations, as well as animals.

- Organic farms use less energy and produce less waste, e.g., packaging materials for chemicals, when calculated either per unit area or per unit of yield.

A 2003 investigation by the UK's Department for Environment Food and Rural Affairs found, similar to other reports, that organic farming "can produce positive environmental benefits." Some of those benefits, however, were decreased or lost when compared on "the basis of unit production rather than area."

Energy Efficiency

A study of the sustainability of apple production systems compared a conventional farming system to an organic farming system. The organic system came out on top as being more energy-efficient.

Safety

Consumer Safety

Widespread belief that organic food is considerably safer to consume than conventionally-grown food has fueled incremented authoritatively mandate for organic food, despite its higher prices. The belief is predicated, mainly, upon anecdotal evidence and testimonials rather than upon scientific evidence. Reviews of the available body of scientific literature comparing the safety of the two has not shown either to be significantly safer than the other. Felicitously appropriate study design and a relatively diminutively minuscule number of studies hampers the ability to reach firm conclusions about organic foods' safety over conventional foods.

Claims of ameliorated safety of organic food has largely centered on pesticide residues. While studies show organically-grown fruits and vegetables contain much lower pesticide residue levels, the significance of this finding on actual health risk reduction is debatable. Generally, pesticide levels in both conventional foods and organic foods is well below regime-established guidelines for what is considered safe. The U.S. Department of Agriculature and the UK Food Standards Agency echo this view. Evidence in medical literature does not support claims of incremented health risks related to pesticide residue and rates of infertility or lower sperm counts. Reviews note that risks from microbiological sources or natural toxins are liable to be much more significant than short-term or chronic risks from pesticide residues.

Focus has been placed on the amount of nitrogen content in certain vegetables, especially green leafy vegetables and tubers, grown organically as compared to conventionally. While these vegetables, when grown organically, have been found to have lower nitrogen content, there is no consensus as to whether consumption of lower levels of nitrogen translates to improved health. When evaluating environmental toxins such as heavy metals, the USDA noted that organically-raised chicken may have lower arsenic levels, while a literature review found no significant evidence that levels of arsenic, or other heavy metals, differed significantly between organic and conventional food products.

Regarding possible increased risk to safety from organic food consumption, reviews show that although theoretical increased risks from microbiological contamination (like *E. coli* 0157:H7) due to increased manure use as fertilizer during organic produce production, insufficient evidence exists of actual outbreaks that can be clearly tied to organic food production to draw any firm conclusions. Other possible sources of increased safety risk from organic food consumption from biological pesticides use, or the theoretical risk from mycotoxins from fungi grown on products due to effective organic-compliant fungicides have likewise not been confirmed by rigorous studies in the scientific literature.

Nutritional Value and Taste

In April 2009, results from Quality Low Input Food (QLIF), a 5-year integrated study funded by the European Commission, confirmed that "the quality of crops and livestock products from organic and conventional farming systems differs considerably." Specifically, results from a QLIF project studying the effects of organic and low-input farming on crop and livestock nutritional quality "showed that organic food production methods resulted, in some cases, to: (a) higher levels of nutritionally-desirable compounds (e.g., vitamins/antioxidants and polyunsaturated fatty acids such as omega-3 and CLA); (b) lower levels of nutritionally-undesirable compounds such as heavy metals, mycotoxins, pesticide residues and glyco-alkaloids in a range of crops and/or milk; (c) a lower risk of faecal Salmonella shedding in pigs." It also showed no significant difference between traditionally grown foods on other studies. The QLIF study also concludes that "further and more detailed studies are required to provide proof for positive health impacts of organic diets on human and animal health." Alternatively, according to the UK's Food Standards Agency, "Consumers may choose to buy organic fruit, vegetables, and meat because they believe them to be more nutritious than other food. However, the balance of current scientific evidence does not support this view." A 12-month systematic review commissioned by the FSA in 2009 and conducted at the London School of Hygiene & Tropical Medicine based on 50 years' worth of collected evidence concluded that "there is no good evidence that consumption of organic food is beneficial to health in relation to nutrient content." Other studies have found no proof that organic food offers greater nutritional values, more consumer safety or any distinguishable difference in taste. A recent review of nutrition claims showed that organic food proponents are unreliable information sources which harm consumers, and that consumers are wasting their money if they buy organic food believing that it contains better nutrients.

Regarding taste, a 2001 study concluded that organic apples were sweeter by blind taste test. Firmness of the apples was also rated higher than those grown conventionally. Current studies have not found differences in the amounts of natural biotoxins between organic and conventional foods.

Economics

Primarily, demand for organic foods is based on concern for personal health and for the environment. Organic products typically cost 10 to 40% more than similar, conventionally-produced products. According to the USDA, Americans, on average, spent $1,347 on groceries in 2004; thus, switching entirely to organics would raise their grocery costs by about $135 to $539 per year ($11 to $45 per month), assuming prices remained stable with increased demand. Processed organic foods vary in price when compared to their conventional counterparts.

While organic food accounts for 1 to 2% of total food sales worldwide, the organic food market is growing rapidly, far ahead of the rest of the food industry, in both developed and developing nations.

Worldwide

- Organic food sales jumped from US $23 billion in 2002 to $52 billion in 2008. The organic market has grown by 20% a year since the early 1990s. Future growth estimates range from 10% to 50% annually, depending on the country.

United States

- Organic food is the fastest growing sector of the American food marketplace.

- Organic food sales have grown by 17 to 20 percent a year for the past few years, while sales of conventional food have grown at about 2 to 3 percent a year.

- In 2003, organic products were available in nearly 20,000 natural food stores and in 73% of conventional grocery stores.

- Organic products accounted for 2.6% of total food sales in the year 2005.

- Two-thirds of organic milk and cream and half of organic cheese and yogurt are sold through conventional supermarkets.

HEALTHY TIP #8: Exercise daily. Start with 5 minutes each day.

The benefits are phenomenal.

REAL MILK

(Bonnie) I'm 53 and have drank real milk most of my life, as my parents, grandparents, great grandparents – generations.

The majority of cows have traditionally been fed grain, corn, and soy-based feeds rather than grass. Therefore, their milk will contain practically none of the conjugated linoleic acid (CLA) that consumers look to as a benefit of drinking milk. Cattle are typically fed growth hormones, used to increase their milk production, and traditionally have been fed antibiotics. The antibiotics are passed along from the cow to the consumer in the milk they drink.

Store-bought milk is pasteurized, meaning it has been heated to at least 145 degrees Fahrenheit. The process, designed to kill off any stray disease-causing bacteria, lamentably kills off the good, lactic acid-producing bacteria die, as well.

Except for skim, all milk is homogenized. This process suspends butterfat, rather than sanctioning it to float to the top. Fat molecules are thereby altered and cause a host of problems, including atherosclerosis.

Drinking real milk helps consumers avoid all of these issues. Yes, drink milk straight from the cow! Raw milk has been demonized as a source of disease, including tuberculosis and anthrax. The truth is quite the opposite: Raw milk contains all the proteins nature has intended to keep our bodies salubrious. Felicitously appropriate handling brings the risk of bacterial contamination to practically zero.

Some farmers are making their raw milk supplies available through share-in-a-dairy-cow programs, in which you share in a portion of the milk. There are no government restrictions on what you can do with your own milk. Look for regional sources for raw milk at www.realmilk.com

If you don't live near a cow-share farmer, or if you prefer the convenience of delivery, contact Organic Pasture Dairy at (977) 729-6455, or visit www. Organicpastures.com. They'll ship their raw milk products anywhere in the US.

HEALTHY TIP #10: Purchase lemon, lime, orange, pine, peppermint or jasmine oils.

Use in potpourri, baths, or just smell the oil.

These oils are all-energizing.

WATER and the HUMAN BODY

HEALTHY TIP #11: Add virgin coconut oil and cold-pressed olive oil to your diet

Both are high in omega oils.

Use coconut oil in your bath water as a moisturizer, and use it on your hair for a great conditioner.

(Bonnie) 75% of Americans are dehydrated, that's a high percentage! I was at an alternative health care seminar a few weeks ago and they are linking dehydration to most illnesses and diseases. When working in my field my first 2 questions to everyone (no mater what their health concerns are) are how much water do you drink and how many ball movements do you have per day? To find out how much water you should have per day, weigh yourself and cut that number in half. That is how many ounces of water you should have every day.

Did you know that

- newborn babies are 77% water as they emerge from the warm and watery solution of their mothers' wombs.
- children are 59% water
- adults are 45% to 65% water

Did you further know that

- the blood is 83% water
- kidneys are 82%
- muscles, 75%
- the brain, 74%
- the liver, 69%
- and bones are 22% water

Water, then, is the principal constituent of fluids surrounding and within all living cells.

Bodily functions heavily dependent upon the presence of water are these:

- respiration,
- digestion,
- assimilations,
- metabolism,
- elimination,
- waste removal,
- and temperature regulation

Water dissolves and transports nutrients, such as oxygen and mineral salts, via the blood, liver, and other body fluids. Water maintains the pressure, acidity, and composition of all chemical reaction in equilibrium.

How We Lose Water

Most water is removed by the kidneys, the organ through which our entire blood supply passes and is filtered 15 times each hour. Amazingly, each time the body overheats, two billion sweat glands activate to excrete perspiration, which is 99 percent water. The blood's heat evaporates the sweat, keeping internal organs at a constant temperature. Perhaps, you're already aware of these ways in which our body sheds water.

However, lesser-known ways in which our body sheds water are through

- breathing and tearing, a minimal but consistent loss
- breathing out moisture from our water-lined nasal passages and lungs. Dry air draws off more water than humid air.
- tearing—a liquid solution carried to tiny tear ducts in the upper eyelids, lubricate the eyes 25 times every minute. Tears passing down to the nose evaporate.

How Lost Water is Replaced

Each day, our bodies require approximately three quarts of water. Exercise, high activity levels, hot temperatures, or diets too high in sodium may increase this amount. The hypothalamus, a part of our forebrains, controls our sense of thirst (and, in addition, controls our sleep, appetite, satiety, and sexual response).

Metabolic water, a byproduct of the food combustion process, yields as much as a pint per day.

Fruits and vegetables, with high water content, add up to one-and-one-half quarts of water, while dry foods, such as bread and crackers, contain 35 and 5 percent water, respectively.

Drinking water is a key method of replenishing it. Many people recommend that we drink six to eight glasses of fresh water every day. These quantities are not only essential for many activities within our bodies; they're critical for most enzymes, as well. Take, for example, the enzymes protease, amylase, and lipase. They're hydrolytic enzymes and require water to activate them so they can do their jobs. Bottom line: Without water, these, and other enzymes, could not function.

Why Water is So Vital

Water accounts for approximately 60 percent of our body weight. Gastric juices, for example, are 99.5 percent water, while our teeth contain just 10 percent water.

So water, the environment necessary for chemical reactions, carries nutrients to each cell, and transports waste from cells. Water helps maintain proper body temperature, whether we're suffering from winter's frozen grip or summer's intense heat. Water provides a protective cushion around the brain and every other body organ.

Summing It All Up

About 60 percent of body water comes from fluids, 30 percent is obtained from foods we eat, and the remaining 10 percent comes from cellular metabolism.

We lose water through perspiration, elimination (in urine and feces), while some water vaporizes from our lungs. When we don't replenish lost water, dehydration results. Signs of dehydration ares: decreased urine output, flushed dry skin; and a very dry mouth. Left unchecked, mental confusion, fever, weight loss, and death can occur.

Water consumption should equal water output if the body is to remain properly hydrated.

Water from most municipal water systems is either contaminated or loaded chemicals. Consider purchasing a good quality water purification system for your home.

(Mary) I was recently at the eye doctor and found out I have dry eyes. I thought I drank a lot of water but the doctor told me to increase the amount. Not only do I feel better, I am taking care of another health concern.

HEALTHY TIP #12: Buy a gratitude journal

Everyday write down 3 things that you are grateful for

NON-FOODS

The benefits of peroxide in place of bleach

HEALTHY TIP #13: Drink green tea daily

It's a great antioxidant, and it's also very alkalizing

(Bonnie) Isn't it great that we always have an alternative? I have a client who ended up with flooding in her basement and I told her about peroxide. She sprayed down the whole basement and it killed the entire mold. Food grade hydrogen peroxide also works great in hot tubs and pools vs chlorine.

When you visit your doctor's office, do you ever smell bleach? Because it not only smells; it's just not healthy. Ask the nurses who work there if they use bleach at home. They know better! Bleach is basically chlorine!

Inside that plain bottle of 3% peroxide that you can buy for less than a dollar at any drugstore, a world of benefits awaits you. What does bleach cost?

Ways to Use Peroxide for Your Good Health:

Mouth Sores: Hold one capful (white bottle cap) in your mouth for 10 minutes daily, then spit it out. No more canker sores! And your teeth will be whiter without expensive pastes. Use it in place of expensive mouthwash.

Toothbrushes: Soak your toothbrushes in a cup of peroxide to keep them free of germs.

Sanitizer: Clean your counters and tabletops with peroxide to kill germs and leave a fresh smell. Simply pour a little onto your dishrag when you wipe, or spray it directly on counters.

Cleaner/Disinfectant: Pour peroxide onto your wooden cutting board after you rinse it off to kill salmonella and other bacteria.

Fungus: Rid yourself of foot fungus. For years, I had fungus on my feet—until I sprayed a 50/50 mixture (peroxide and water) on them, especially between the toes, every night, then I let them dry.

Infections: Soak infections or cuts in 3% peroxide for 5 to 10 minutes several times a day. My husband has seen gangrene that would not heal with any medicine but did heal by soaking in peroxide.

Bath and Shower Cleaner: Keep a spray bottle filled with a 50/50 mixture of peroxide and water in every bathroom. It disinfects without harming your septic system as will bleach and most other disinfectants.

Colds, Sinuses and Infections: Tilt your head back and spray a 50/50 mixture into nostrils at the first sign of a cold or plugged sinuses. The bubbling action is killing offending bacteria. Hold for several minutes, then blow your nose gently into a tissue.

Natural Hair Highlighter: Spray the 50/50 solution onto wet hair and comb it through for natural highlights, if your hair is light-brown, reddish, or dirty blonde. You'll avoid the peroxide-burnt blonde look that comes from using packaged hair dye. Since the mixture lightens gradually, you'll also avoid a harsh and drastic change.

Infections: Use one-half bottle of peroxide in your bath to eliminate boils, fungus, or other skin infections.

Laundry: Add a cup of peroxide instead of bleach to a load of whites on laundry day to whiten your clothes. For bloodstains, pour peroxide directly onto the soiled area. Let sit for a minute, then rub it. Rinse with cold water. Repeat, if necessary.

Windows and Mirrors: Clean mirrors with peroxide. It leaves no smearing, a reason why I love it so much for this household cleaning task.

There are many more options for using peroxide. With prices of most necessities constantly on the rise, I'm glad there's a way to save so much money, so simply!

HEALTHY TIP # 14: Eat more live, raw food

RADIATION DETOX BATH

(Bonnie) I recommend everyone do the radiation detox baths, greens, seaweeds, foods, herbs and supplements and diets at least 2 times per year. We are all exposed to radiation, power lines, towers, cell phones and computers. Doing the detox is just a great precautionary medicine.

At home

It's possible, right in your own home, to help your body heal from radiation exposure. **You can also help your body heal by excreting and keeping the organs of elimination open.**

I'm presuming the emergency or exposure is over, and you're looking for ways to detox yourself from months, even years, of contamination. As you know by now, our skin is our body's major organ of elimination. To pull heavy metal toxins out of your skin, take a therapeutic bath, which is another form of detox cleansing.

How to bathe out toxins

First, bear these things in mind: Hot water followed by cold water bathing increases circulation. Toxins are drawn to the skin's surface because of the change in temperature. To benefit from this type of therapeutic healing, it's **essential** that you remain in the bathwater through the cooldown.

The Epson Salt Bath

Fill your bathtub with water as hot as you can tolerate. Add and let dissolve one pound of sea salt or rock salt and one pound of baking soda. Now, soak in the water until it has cooled. This may take 20 and 25 minutes. Do not shower or rinse the salt off your body for 4 to 8 hours after the bath.

For Extra Exposure

If you've been exposed to atmospheric, low-grade radioactive materials, dissolve two pounds of baking soda in a tub of hot water. As above, stay in the water until it has cooled.

While taking this type of bath, sip green tea and herbal teas, or alkalize your body by sipping a mixture of one-half teaspoon baking soda in a glass of warm water.

Nighttime, the time when the body is geared to detoxification, is the best time for this type of bathing. Take only one bath per day.

Continue the detoxification baths until you feel relief from radiation symptoms. Use common sense, however, and cut back or discontinue them if they are too strong or unpleasant. Symptoms to watch for are vomiting, diarrhea, headache, and fatigue.

These baths are harmless, and do not damage the body, and a number of doctors and naturopaths recommend them. Why? Because radioactive contaminants are heavy metals, and baths help the skin shed excess heavy metals. We're all exposed in some way to exposure from nuclear testing, nuclear accidents, and leaks from nuclear power plants—through the air we breath, the food we eat, and the water we drink.

Clay Baths

Clay draws heavy metals from the skin, and radioactive metals are the heaviest metals of all. Any type of internal or external detoxification routine will prove useful for radiation detoxification, though some protocols will be more effective than others. (See section below, **Bathable and Edible Clays**.)

Spirulina, Chlorella, and Seaweed

When the Chernobyl (Ukraine) reactor meltdown disaster struck in 1986, approximately 134 plant workers and firefighters battling the fire at the plant were exposed to high doses of radiation—80,000 to 1,600,000 mrem (800 to 16,000 mSv)—and suffered from acute radiation sickness. In the first few days after the meltdown, two patients died from their radiation injuries. Within the first three months, 28 more died.

In total, victims of radiation poisoning numbered over 160,000 children and 146,000 cleanup workers. The radiation produced a higher incidence of birth defects, leukemia, anemia, cancers, thyroid disease, spinal fluid degeneration, liver, and bone marrow cancers, and severely compromised immune systems.

The Institute of Radiation Medicine in Minsk found that, by taking **5 grams of spirulina a day for 45 days**, the children showed enhanced immune systems and T-cell counts, along with *reduced radioactivity*.

We don't really know why or how consuming spirulina protects the human body from radiation. We just know that it works. One aspect of spirulina to be considered is its high beta carotene content which reduces free radical damage to cells. It's even been used to treat cancer.

Spirulina

- o   is extremely rich in highly-bioavailable iron, and helps build the blood in anemia patients. Anemia makes up a significant portion of radiation sickness.

- o   is of great benefit to malnutrition patients suffering radiation sickness.

- o   is chockfull of nutrients, it's highly digestible, and helps the body absorb nutrients while the body is weakest.

- o   staves off malnutrition and allows the body to absorb food more effectively.

- o   and other algae contain high amounts of metallothionine compounds, which may strip the body of radioactive metals and protect against radiation damage.

- o   should become part of the standard diet because of its healing benefits.

Kidneys are among the first organs to suffer damage from radiation toxicity. Research suggests that, when spirulina is added to an anti-cancer, antibiotic, painkilling drug protocol, toxic side effects can be significantly reduced, and shorter recovery times may be possible.

Sea Vegetables

There is no family of foods more protective against radiation and environmental pollutants than sea vegetables, which can prevent assimilation of radionucleotides, heavy metals such as cadmium, and other environmental toxins.

Sea vegetables are 10 to 20 times higher in vitamins, minerals, and amino acids than land-grown plants. By its absorbability alone, those dietary benefits make them ideal foods for anyone suffering from radiation sickness.

Kelp

Kelp are the longest of the sea plants. They're thicker, darker yellow-brown seaweeds, known as the brown seaweeds. In China and Japan, kelp is used to treat thyroid problems. Their alginic acid, absorbs toxic elements out of the body. Use these tasty delicacies in any soup.

Chlorella

Chlorella is, honestly, a natural wonder food, and the most researched algae in the world. Countless studies show it has a **radioprotective effect** on gamma ray-induced chromosomal damage, while possessing anti-tumor properties.

Chlorella builds the immune system, detoxifies heavy metals, normalizes blood sugar and blood pressure, balances the body's pH, fights cancer, and protects against ultraviolet radiation. Due to its high chlorophyll content, it helps detoxify the liver, bowel, and bloodstream.

A chlorophyll-rich diet has been shown to increase the survival of experimental animals after they were given lethal doses of radiation.

Chlorella and other algae are also abundant in beta-carotene. The substance is known to prevent cancer and fight cancer by using high doses of chlorella.

Several years ago, Japanese doctors also discovered that giving chlorella to cancer patients undergoing radiation therapy helped **prevent leucopenia**, the sudden drop in white blood cell count, and a major problem with radiation illness! By giving chlorella in advance of the radiation (or chemotherapy) treatment, doctors found that white blood cell count did not drop as low, and bounced back toward normal more quickly than usual. Since chlorella is not found in foods (it is an algae grown in fresh water), take in capsule powder, pill, or tincture form.

Bathable and Edible Clays for Radiation Detox

Clays are particularly known for their ability to remove toxic metals from the air, water, and soil because of their unusual "pore" structure (channels and holes) that allow them to absorb huge amounts of contaminant materials. Therefore, their unique structure gives clays unusual filtering capabilities for absorbing toxic wastes, including radioactive contaminants.

It's been reported that 40 percent of an edible purified zeolite product like **Natural Cellular Defense** binds the heavy metals in the gastrointestinal tract, while 60 percent binds toxins in the bloodstream. At the Chernobyl disaster site, the crystalline structure of zeolites was used to trap and remove radioactive cesium and strontium-90 from affected individuals' systems.

While you can take an Epson salt bath, you can also take a detox bath of zeolite clay specially formulated with special herbs for this purpose. Find order information for the **Zeo-rad Detox Bath,** which contains zeolite clay, at www.blessedbaths.com.

Bentonite clay absorbs heavy metals and contaminants in the intestine, and is often part of colon cleansing routines. **Liquid Bentonite** (hydrated bentonite) is available in health food stores. There are more than 200 different types of bentonite clay. Some contain extremely high amounts of aluminum. For that reason, do not ingest them on a *frequent basis*. Years ago, the same high alumina content problem existed with various colloidal mineral solutions, chockfull of heavy metals. I had spectroscopic studies performed on a number of them, and found the alumina contents were off the charts!

Bentonite **adsorbs** radiation so well that it was the material dumped on top of the Chernobyl nuclear power plant after that nuclear meltdown.

LL's Magnetic Clay Baths has a superior **Environmental Detox Bath** useful for heavy metal detox. It's also useful in removing radiation. This product is composed of **bentonite clay** and contains under .5% aluminum and no emulsifiers.

As with all clays, the more you use them, the quicker you'll detox.

The **Environmental Detox Bath** is another possibility for any heavy metal detoxification routine you decide to undertake, and is actually stronger than **Zeo-rad Bath**. Take this type of general-purpose detoxification bath just once a week for 6 to 10 weeks.

Eat A "Nucleotide Rich" Diet to Maximize Cellular Repair

What are nucleotides? They're the building blocks or sub-unit molecules that make up RNA and DNA, which carry your genetic code. Nucleotides also carry out several essential functions needed for cell replication. They perform the following functions in your body:

- Neutralize toxins
- Increase cellular metabolism
- Increase production of cellular energy
- Improve response and efficiency of the immune system
- Enhance the effects of antioxidants
- Increase the body's ability to heal and repair

Foods, Herbs and Supplements That Are "Radio-Protective"

To help RNA/DNA repair (and post-radiation exposure would be one such instance where you'll want this help), it makes sense to include foods in your diet that contain abundant levels -- and I mean *really abundant* levels -- of nucleotides since they are the building blocks from which your body builds DNA and RNA.

Most importantly, however, are the foods that contain large portions of nucleic acids: sea algae (like chlorella and spirulina), liver, nutritional yeast, bee pollen.

- **Spirulina** (blue-green algae), chlorella (a green algae), liver, nutritional yeast, bee pollen contain large portions of nucleic acids. Brewer's yeast, lentils, most beans, oysters, sardines, anchovies, and mackerel are all known for their healthy, anti-aging, and repairing characteristics

- **Juicing fruits and vegetables** is another remedy for radically healing the body. They contain high concentrations of nucleotides.

- **Black and green tea** have shown to possess radio-protective effects, whether consumed before or *after* exposure to radiation. This anti-radiation effect was observed in several Japanese studies. Chinese studies also suggest that the ingredients in tea are radioactive antagonists. One reason tea offers anti-radiation effects similar to seaweeds is its catechins. They absorb radioactive isotopes and remove them from the body, just like the active ingredient *sodium alginate* in kelp seaweed. Epigallo-catechin-gallate (EGCG), found in some green tea extracts, has also been shown to protect body cells against the free radical damage caused by radioactivity. Black and green tea help against cancer.

In other words, much like seaweed, the ingredients in green tea absorb radioactive isotopes so the body excretes them. They also contain the cancer-fighting compound EGCG.

- Red tea, **Rooibos,** contains the flavonoid compound **luteolin**, and is effective in withstanding radiation.

Source: Top Shape Publishing LLC, *MediationExpert.com*. Radiation Detox

< http://www.meditationexpert.com/RadiationDetoxDraft.pdf>

A High-Fiber and Mineral-Rich Diet

To deter absorption of radioactive particles and improve their excretion, a high-fiber diet of easily-digested vegetables (but no produce exposed to radiation fallout) makes sense and is recommended. The purpose behind eating clay, kelp, and pectin is to bind radionuclides in the gut. A high-fiber diet accomplishes the same thing.

Because they also aid in the excretion of radioactive particles, supplements high in calcium and potassium, particularly cesium-137 are foods you'll want to eat. You can also take them in supplement form.

Selenium (found in yeast), in particular, has been shown to protect human DNA from radiation damage and helps prevent skin damage, too. Green and black teas, garlic, many types of mushrooms, such as button and shiitake mushrooms, are good sources of selenium. However, the best sources are **nettles** (2200 mcg per 100 grams), **kelp** (1700 mcg/100 g), **burdock** (1400 mcg/100 g), **catnip** (Nepeta cataria), **ginseng, Siberian ginseng**, and **astragalus**.

Seaweeds, along with spirulina and chlorella, are an easily digestible, absorbable form of selenium.

Consume More Lycopene and Foods Rich in Beta-Carotene

Another food to add to the diet after radiation exposure is cooked tomato sauce because of its high lycopene content. **Lycopene**, which gives tomatoes their red color, has been shown to protect against cancer formation, prevents the destructive and mutagenic effects of gamma radiation, and protects against the effects of ultraviolet irradiation of the skin. It is a carotenoid and like other carotenoids, lycopene enhances general immunity. It may be particularly effective in improving the action of T-cells and inhibiting cancer.

Eat More from the Cabbage Family and Sulphur-Containing Compounds

The brassica family of foods is particularly beneficial for their radio-protective effects, and their ability to repair radiation damage. Eat daily from this food family: Cabbage, broccoli, cauliflower, Brussels Sprouts, kale, collards, arugula, turnips, radishes, mustard greens, bok choy.

Add Dried Beans or Lentils to Your Diet

Do you remember that dried beans, especially lentils, were in that short list of foods rich in nucleotides? *** Studies have indeed proved they can reverse DNA damage caused by radiation. It's yet another reason to include them as part of the anti-radiation diet.

Three members of the legume (bean) family -- **lentils**, **red clover** (*Trifolium pratense*), and **astragalus** (*Astragalus membranaceous*) -- are well-known for their anti-radiation and cancer-fighting effects and help reverse the damaging effects of radiation. Astragalus is an ingredient found in most Chinese strengthening formulas.

Nutritionists commonly advise cancer patients to drink red clover tea, and to take astragalus supplements. However, their exact use is outside the scope of this discussion. While it is the beans, in general, that I want you to concentrate on, I want you to know about these other two members of the bean family used for anti-cancer purposes.

Eat Red Beets

Exposure to radiation can affect your body's ability to produce red blood cells. A well-known American holistic remedy (Europeans also use it) for quickly rebuilding the blood and fighting anemia is to drink raw or fermented **beet juice** which helps build blood hemoglobin. Consuming beet root is a natural remedy for nerve cell inflammation, and another bonus in repairing the nervous system from severe radiation exposure.

Reishi Mushrooms, Glucans and Polysaccharides to Bolster Immune Health

Time for mushrooms.

Eating Reishi mushrooms is a proven way to reduce damage from radiation and to bolster the immune system after radiation exposure. They *slowly* boost the immune system, a wise course of action after radiation exposure. The mushrooms of choice are Reishi and Coriolus (which fight cancer), though consider eating **Cat's Claw***** which is known for its ability to prevent damage to DNA and repair damaged DNA. **Thymus extract** is also a well-known immunological stimulant.

Aloe Vera for Radiation Burns and Healing

Aloe Vera has a long history of treating serious radiation burns. It offers radioprotective effects. Apply it to skin, or ingest it.

Various Herbs

Burdock root,*** used as a blood purifier for centuries, is said to remove radioactive isotopes from the body as part of its ability to neutralize and eliminate poisons from the body. It has also been included in the famous Hoxsey formula, and Rene Caisse's Essiac cancer formulas. Essiac tea, by the way, is a famous cancer preventative whose constituents (burdock root, sheep sorrel, slippery elm bark, turkey rhubarb root) clean the body and help dissolve tumors.

Burdock also supports the bladder, kidney and liver. It contains niacin, along with an abundance of minerals, particularly iron.

Turmeric*** contains **curcumin**, an ingredient that gives curry and mustard its yellow color. It is said to substantially decrease the damaging effects of radiation.

*** We carry Red Clover tincture and astragalus tincture, and Cat's Claw; and we carry burdock, and turmeric.

HEALTHY TIP #15: Listen to music that makes you want to swing your hips

Let go of anger, fear, and resentment

CHARTS & GUIDES

COMMON FOODS and THEIR HEALTH BENEFITS

HEALTHY TIP #16: Volunteer – It will bring you an awareness and appreciation for your own life

If you don't have the time to volunteer, help someone every day

Apples:	Apricots:
• Protect the heart • Improve lung capacity • Prevent constipation • Cushion joints	• Combat cancer • Shield against Alzheimer's • Control blood pressure • Slow aging • Save eyesight
Artichokes:	Avocadoes:
• Aid digestion • Stabilize blood sugars • Lower cholesterol • Guard against liver disease • Protect the heart	• Battle diabetes • Control blood pressure • Lower cholesterol • Smooth skin • Help stop strokes
Bananas:	Beans:
• Protect the heart • Control blood pressure • Quiet a cough • Block diarrhea • Strengthen bones	• Prevent constipation • Combat cancer • Help hemorrhoids • Stabilize blood sugar • Lower cholesterol

Beets:	Blueberries:
• Control blood pressure • Protect the heart • Combat cancer • Aid weight loss • Strengthen bones	• Combat cancer • Boost memory • Protect the heart • Prevent constipation • Stabilize blood sugar
Broccoli:	**Cabbage:**
• Strengthens bones • Protects the heart • Saves eyesight • Controls blood pressure • Combats cancer	• Combats cancer • Protects the heart • Prevents constipation • Helps hemorrhoids • Promotes weight loss
Cantaloupe:	**Carrots:**
• Saves eyesight • Combats cancer • Controls blood pressure • Supports immune system • Lowers cholesterol	• Save eyesight • Prevent constipation • Protect the heart • Promote weight loss
Cauliflower:	**Cherries**
• Protects against prostate cancer • Banishes bruises • Combats breast cancer • Guards against heart disease • Strengthens bones	• Protect the heart • Slow aging • Combat cancer • Shield against Alzheimer's • End insomnia

Chestnuts:	Chili Peppers:
• Promote weight loss • Combat cancer • Protect the heart • Control blood pressure • Lower cholesterol	• Aid digestion • Combat cancer • Soothe sore throat • Boost immune system • Clear sinuses
Figs:	Fish:
• Promote weight loss • Combat cancer • Help stop strokes • Control blood pressure • Lower cholesterol	• Protects the heart • Combats cancer • Boosts memory • Supports immune system • Protects the heart
Flax:	Garlic:
• Aids digestion • Improves mental health • Battles diabetes • Boosts immune system • Protects the heart	• Lowers cholesterol • Kills bacteria • Controls blood pressure • Fights fungus • Combats cancer
Grapefruit:	Grapes:
• Protects against heart attacks • Combats prostrate cancer • Promotes weight loss • Lowers cholesterol • Helps stop strokes	• Save eyesight • Enhance blood flow • Conquer kidney stones • Protect the heart • Combat cancer

Green Tea:	Honey:
• Combats cancer • Promotes weight loss • Protects the heart • Kills bacteria • Helps stop strokes	• Heals wounds • Increases energy • Aids digestion • Fights allergies • Guards against ulcers
Lemons:	Limes:
• Combat cancer • Smooth skin • Protect the heart • Stop scurvy • Control blood pressure	• Combat cancer • Smooth skin • Protect the heart • Stop scurvy • Control blood pressure
Mangoes:	Mushrooms:
• Combat cancer • Aid digestion • Boost memory • Shield against Alzheimer's • Regulate thyroid	• Control blood pressure • Combat cancer • Lower cholesterol • Strengthen bones • Kill bacteria
Oats:	Olive oil:
• Lower cholesterol • Prevent constipation • Combat cancer • Smooth skin • Battle diabetes	• Protects the heart • Battles diabetes • Promotes weight loss • Smoothes skin • Combats cancer

Onions:	Oranges:
<ul><li>Reduce risk of heart attack</li><li>Lower cholesterol</li><li>Combat cancer</li><li>Fight fungus</li><li>Kill bacteria</li></ul>	<ul><li>Support immune systems</li><li>Protect the heart</li><li>Combat cancer</li><li>Strengthen respiration</li></ul>
Peaches:	Peanuts:
<ul><li>Prevent constipation</li><li>Aid digestion</li><li>Combat cancer</li><li>Help hemorrhoids</li><li>Help stop strokes</li></ul>	<ul><li>Protect against heart disease</li><li>Lower cholesterol</li><li>Promote weight loss</li><li>Aggravate diverticulitis</li><li>Combat prostate cancer</li></ul>

Pineapple:	Prunes:
• Strengthens bones • Dissolves warts • Relieves colds • Blocks diarrhea • Aids digestion	• Slow aging • Lower cholesterol • Prevent constipation • Protect against heart disease • Boost memory
Rice:	Strawberries:
• Protects the heart • Combats cancer • Battles diabetes • Helps stop strokes • Conquers kidney stones	• Combat cancer • Boost memory • Protect the heart • Calm stress
Sweet potatoes:	Tomatoes:
• Save eyesight • Combat cancer • Lift mood • Strengthen bones	• Protect prostate • Lower cholesterol • Combat cancer • Protect the heart
Walnuts:	Water:
• Lower cholesterol • Lift moods • Combat cancer • Protect against heart disease • Boost memory	• Promotes weight loss • Conquers kidney stones • Combats cancer • Smoothes skin

Watermelon:	Wheat germ:
• Protects prostate • Helps stop strokes • Promotes weight loss • Controls blood pressure • Lowers cholesterol	• Combats colon cancer • Helps stop strokes • Prevents constipation • Improves digestion • Lowers cholesterol
Wheat bran:	Yogurt:
• Combats colon cancer • Helps stop strokes • Prevents constipation • Improves digestion • Lowers cholesterol	• Guards against ulcers • Supports immune system • Strengthens bones • Aids digestion • Lowers cholesterol

HEALTHY TIP #17: Pray, meditate, follow your spirit

Do something you loved doing as a child

Play in the rain or snow

NATURAL SUPPLEMENT GUIDE: A Complete Guide to Vitamins, Minerals, and Herbs

Vitamin	Natural Sources	Affected Components
Vitamin A	Alfalfa, Beef, Beets, Burdock, Butter, Carrots, Cayenne, Cheese and Other Dairy Products, Chicken Liver, Cod Liver Oil, Colorado Fruits, Dandelion, Fish Liver Oils Garlic, Green Leafy Vegetables (Kale, Turnip Greens, Spinach), Kelp, Marshmallow, Melon, Papaya, Parsley, Pokeweed, Raspberry, Red Clover, Saffron, Spirulina, Squash, Tomatoes, Watercress, Yams, Yellow Dock	Adrenal Glands, Bones, Eyes, Hair, Immune System, Mucous Linings and Membranes, Nails, Skin Cells, Teeth
Vitamin B1 - Thiamine	Asparagus, Beets, Brewer's Yeast, Cayenne, Dandelion, Egg Yolks, Fenugreek, Fish, Kelp, Leafy Green Vegetables, Liver, Milk and Dairy Products, Nuts and Nut Butters, Oatmeal, Parsley, Plums, Potatoes, Poultry, Prunes, Raisins, Raspberry, Rice Polishings, Seeds (All), Soybeans, Wheat Germ	Brain, Ears, Eyes, Hair, Heart, Muscles, Nervous System

Vitamin B2 – Riboflavin	Alfalfa, Almonds, Asparagus, Beef Liver and Kidney, Brewer's Yeast, Broccoli, Burdock, Cheese and Other Dairy Products, Cooked Leafy Vegetables, Currants, Dandelion, Egg Yolks, Enriched Cereals and Breads, Fenugreek, Fish, Kelp, Milk, Parsley, Raspberry, Sunflower Seeds, Torula Yeast, Wheat Germ, Whole Grains, Yogurt	Eyes, Hair, Nails, Skin
Vitamin B3 – Niacin	Alfalfa, Avocados, Burdock, Brewer's Yeast, Dandelion, Dates, Egg, Fenugreek, Figs, Fish, Green Vegetables, Kelp, Kidney, Lean Meat, Liver, Parsley, Prunes, Rice Bran, Rice Polishings, Roasted Peanuts, Sage, Sunflower Seeds, Torula Yeast, Wheat Germ, White Meat of Poultry, Whole Wheat Products	Brain, Gastro-intestinal Tract, Heart, Liver, Nervous System, Sexual Organs, Skin
Vitamin B5 – Pantothenic Acid	Beef, Brewers Yeast, Brown Rice, Cauliflower, Crude Molasses, Egg Yolk, Green Vegetables, Kale, Kidney, Liver, Peas and Beans, Peanuts, Pork, Royal Jelly, Saltwater Fish, Sweet Potatoes, Wheat Bran, Wheat Germ, Whole Grain Breads and Cereals	Adrenal Glands, Brain, Digestive Systems, Immune System, Skin

Vitamin B6 – Pyridoxine	Alfalfa, Avocados, Bananas, Beef, Blackstrap Molasses, Brewer's Yeast, Cantaloupe, Carrots, Corn, Eggs, Green Leafy Vegetables, Green Peppers, Heart, Herring, Kidney, Liver, Milk, Mugwort, Peanuts, Pecans, Soybeans, Salmon, Walnuts, Wheat, Wheat Bran, Wheat Germ	Blood, Muscles, Nerves, Skin

Vitamin B9 – Folic Acid	Asparagus, Beef, Pork Liver, and Kidney, Beet Greens, Brewer's Yeast, Broccoli, Deep Green Leafy Vegetables, Lettuce, Lima Beans, Mushrooms, Nuts, Salmon, Spinach, Sweet Potatoes, Wheat Germ, Whole Wheat	Blood, Cells, Hair, Liver and Skin, Lymph Glands
Vitamin B12 – Cobalamine	Alfalfa, Bananas, Bee Pollen, Beef, Brewer's Yeast, Cheese, Clams, Comfrey Leaves, Concord Grapes, Crab, Egg Yolks, Kelp, Lamb and Beef Kidney, Liver, Milk, Oysters, Peanuts, Pork, Salmon, Sardines, Sunflower Seeds, Wheat Germ	Brain, Nervous System, Red Blood Cells
Vitamin B13 – Orotic Acid	Root Vegetables, The Liquid Portion of Soured or Curdled Milk, Whey	Cells, Liver
Vitamin B15 – Calcium Pangamate	Brewer's Yeast, Nuts, Pumpkin Seeds, Sesame Seeds, Whole Brown Rice, Whole Grains	Glands, Heart Kidneys, Nerves

Vitamin B17 – Laetrile Nitrilosides	Apricots, Blackberries, Blueberries, Cranberries, Flaxseed, Garbanzo, Lima Beans, Mung Beans, Peach and Plum Pits, Raspberries, Whole Seeds	Not known
Vitamin C – Ascorbic Acid	Alfalfa, Apples, Beet Greens, Black Currants, Burdock, Boneset, Broccoli, Brussels Sprouts, Cabbage, Catnip, Cauliflower, Cayenne, Chickweed, Chives, Citrus Fruits, Collards, Dandelion, Garlic, Lima Beans, Guavas, Hawthorn Berry, Horseradish, Kale, Kelp, Kohlrabi, Lobelia, Papaya, Parsley, Peppers, Persimmons, Plantain, Pokeweed, Raspberry, Rose Hips, Shepard's Purse, Spinach, Squash, Strawberry, Sweet Potatoes, Swiss Chard, Tomatoes, Turnip Greens, Watercress, Yellow Dock	Adrenal Glands, Blood, Bones, Capillary Walls, Gums, Heart, Ligaments, Skin, Teeth
Vitamin D – Ergosterol	Alfalfa, Butter, Egg Yolks, Fish Oils, Halibut, Herring, Milk, Mushrooms, Salmon, Sardines, Sea Bass, Sprouted Seeds, Sunflower Seeds, Sweet Potatoes, Swordfish, Tuna, Watercress	Bones, Heart, Nerves, Skin, Teeth, Thyroid Gland

Vitamin E	Alfalfa, Brown Rice Nuts, Brussels Sprouts, Corn, Dairy Products, Dandelion, Egg Yolks, Kelp, Leafy Dark Green Vegetables, Raspberry, Red Meats, Rose Hips, Safflower, Soybeans, Spinach, Watercress, Wheat Germ, Whole Wheat, Whole Wheat Products	Adrenal Glands, Blood Vessels, Heart, Liver, Lungs, Pituitary Glands, Skin, Testes, Uterus

Vitamin F	Almonds, Avocados, Cod, Mackerel, Parsley, Peanuts, Safflower, Herring, Salmon, Shrimp, Soybeans, Sunflower Seeds, Tuna, Walnuts, Wheat Germ	Adrenal Glands, Arteries, Cells, Hair, Heart, Nerves, Skin, Thyroid Glands
Vitamin H – Biotin	Beef, Brewer's Yeast, Chicken, Egg Yolk, Fruits, Kidney, Lamb, Milk, Nuts, Pork, Saltwater Fish, Soybeans, Unpolished Rice, Veal Liver, Whole Wheat Flour	Hair, Muscles, Skin
Vitamin K – Menadione	Alfalfa, Beef Liver, Cheese, Egg Yolk, Fish Liver Oil, Kelp, Leafy Green Vegetables, Plantain, Safflower and Soybean Oil, Shepard's Purse, Tomatoes, Turnip Greens, Vegetable Oils, Whole Wheat, Yogurt	Blood, Bones, Capillary Walls, Gums, Ligaments, Skin, Teeth
Vitamin P – Rutin	Apricots, Blackberries, Blueberries, Buckwheat, the White Skins and Segment Parts of all Citrus Fruit, Cherries, Dandelion, Grapeseed Extract, Rose Hips, Rue, Saskatoon Berries	Blood, Bones, Capillary Walls, Gums, Ligaments, Skin, Teeth
Vitamin T	Egg Yolks, Sesame Butter, Sesame Seeds	Blood
Vitamin U	Fresh Cabbage, Raw Cabbage Juice, Sauerkraut	Stomach
Boron	Beets and Beet Tops, Carrots, Fruits, Leafy Vegetables, Legumes, Nuts, Parsnips, Potatoes, Saltwater Fish, Summer Squash, Tomatoes, Whole Grain	Bones, Muscles

| Calcium | Agar, Almonds, Asparagus, Avocados, Barley, Beet Greens, Beans, Blackstrap Molasses, Bran, Brazil Nuts, Broccoli, Brown Rice, Brussels Sprouts, Buckwheat, Butter (Raw), Cabbage, Caraway Seed, Carob, Carrots, Cauliflower, Cheese, Chive, Chamomile, Clams, Cleavers, Coltsfoot, Coconut, Cornmeal (Yellow), Dairy Produce, Dandelion, Dark Leafy Vegetables, Dill, Dulse, Eggs, Figs, Fish, Gelatin, Greens, Horsetail, Irish Moss, Kale, Kelp, Kohlrabi, Lentils, Meadow Sweet, Milk, Millet, Mistletoe, Navy Beans, Nettles, Oats, Onions, Oysters, Parsley, Peanuts, Plantain, Poppy Seed, Prunes, Raspberry, Rye, Salmon, Sardines, Sesame Seeds, Shepard's Purse, Silverweed, Soybeans, Sunflower Seeds, Tofu, Tortillas, Walnuts, Watercress, Wheat, Yellow Dock | Blood, Bones, Heart, Nails, Skin, Soft Tissue, Teeth |

Chlorine	Alfalfa, Asparagus, Avocado, Banana, Beans, Beets, Blackberries, Brazil Nuts, Brussels Sprouts, Cabbage, Carrots, Cauliflower, Celery, Chard, Chives, Coconut, Corn, Cucumber, Dandelion, Dates, Dill Stems, Eggplant, Fennel Stems, Figs, Fish, Fowl, Goat's Milk (Raw), Goldenseal, Horseradish, Kale, Kelp, Kohlrabi, Lean Meat, Leeks, Lentils, Lettuce Leaf, Mango, Nettles, Oats, Olives, Parsley, Parsnip, Peaches, Peas, Pineapple, Plantain, Potatoes with Skins, Radishes, Raisins, Raspberry, Rutabaga, Sauerkraut, Spinach, Strawberries, Sunflower, Seeds, Sweet Potatoes, Tomatoes, Turnips, Uva Ursi, Watercress, Watermelon, Wintergreen	Blood, Cells, Liver, Stomach
Chlorophyll	Alfalfa, Most Leafy Green Potherbs	Tissue Blood
Chromium	Brewer's Yeast, Cane Sugar, Cheese, Chicken, Clams, Dried Beans, Meat, Shellfish, Potatoes, Sunflower and Corn Oil, Whole Grain Cereals	Arteries, Blood, Heart
Cobalt	Beef or Pork Kidney and Liver, Clams, Green Leafy Vegetables, Lean Red Meat, Milk, Oysters, Poultry, Saltwater Fish	Blood, Bones, Brain, Connective Tissues, Heart, Kidney, Liver, Nerves

Fluorine	Avocados, Black-Eyed Peas, Brussels Sprouts, Cabbage, Caraway seeds, Cauliflower, Dates, Eggs, Goat Butter, Cream (Raw), Greens, Juniper Berries, Lemon Grass, Licorice, Parsley, Rye Bran or Meal, Spinach, Tomatoes	Bones, Teeth
Iodine	Agar, Bass, Beans (Butter, French, Kidney, Snap), Blueberries, Brussels Sprouts, Cardamom, Carrot, Chives, Coconut, Cucumber, Eggplant, Fish, Goat Cottage Cheese, Goat Milk, Green Peppers, Haddock, Halibut, Herring, Kale, Leaf Lettuce, Loganberries, Oats, Steel Cut, Okra, Onion, Peanuts, Sweet Potatoes, Quail, Rutabaga, Seaweed, Sole, Strawberries, Tofu, Tune, Tomatoes, Watermelon	Brain, Hair, Nails, Skin, Teeth, Thyroid Gland
Iron	Agar, Almonds, Beet Greens, Blackberry, Black Walnuts, Butternuts, Cashews, Dates, Dried Fruits, Fennel, Figs, Goat Milk, Kale, Lentils (Dried), Millet, Mung Beans, Peas (Dried), Pumpkin Seeds, Radishes, Red Beans, Red Peppers, Rice Polishings and Bran, Rye, Sorrel, Soybeans (Dried), Spinach, Sprouted Seeds, Sunflower Seeds	Blood, Bones, Nails, Skin, Teeth

Magnesium	Agar, Alfalfa, Almonds, Apples, Apricots, Avocados, Bananas (Dried), Beet Tops, Blue Cohosh, Brazil Nuts, Brewer's Yeast, Brown Rice, Burdock, Cabbage, Carrot Leaves, Cashews, Cayenne, Celery, Chard, Coconut, Comfrey Leaves, Corn, Cornmeal (Yellow), Dandelion, Dates, Dill, Dulse, Figs, Fish, Gelatin, Grapes, Green Peppers, Goat Milk, Hickory Nuts, Honey, Kale, Kelp, Lemons, Lentils, Liver, Mistletoe, Mullein, Nettles, Nuts, Oats, Okra, Parsley, Peaches, Peas (Dried), Peanuts, Pears, Pecans, Peppermint, Primrose, Prunes, Rice (Wild or Brown), Rye, Salmon, Sesame Seeds, Sorrell, Spinach, Tofu, Turnip Greens, Walnut Leaves, Watercress, Whole Grains, Whole Wheat, Willow, Wintergreen, Yellow Corn	Arteries, Bones, Blood, Heart, Muscles, Nerves, Teeth
Manganese	Apricots, Bananas, Beets and Beet Leaves, Blackberries, Black-Eyed Peas, Blueberries, Brussels Sprouts, Butternuts, Cardamom, Chestnuts, Citrus Fruits, Egg Yolks, Kelp, Mint, Nuts, Oats (Steel Cut), Parsley, Peas, Pineapple, Rye Meal, Walnuts, Spinach, Tea, Wheat Germ, Whole Grains	Brain, Muscles, Nerves, Thyroid

Molybdenum	Brewer's Yeast, Brown Rice, Buckwheat, Leafy Vegetables, Legumes, Millet, Whole Grain Cereals	Blood
Phosphorus	Alfalfa, Almonds, Barley, Bass, Beans (Lima, Red), Blue Cohosh, Bone Broth, Cabbage, Calendula, Canned Fish, Caraway, Cardamom, Carrots, Cashews, Cayenne, Cereals, Cheese (Swiss), Chickweed, Cod, Corn, Dairy Products (Raw), Dandelion, Dried Fruits, Dulse, Egg, Egg Yolk, Garlic, Goat Butter, Haddock, Halibut, Hard Cheeses, Herring, Irish Moss, Kelp, Legumes, Licorice, Meat, Milk (Raw) and Other Dairy Products, Millet, Oats, Olives (Ripe), Parsley, Pecans, Purslane, Pokeweed, Poultry, Pumpkin Seeds, Raspberry, Rhubarb, Rose Hips, Seeds and Nuts, Walnuts, Watercress, Wheat Germ, Whole Grains, Yeast, Yellow Dock	Bones, Brain, Cell Walls, Heat, Kidneys, Nerves, Teeth

| Potassium | Alfalfa, Almonds, Anise Seed, Apples, Apple Cider Vinegar, Apricots (Dried), Bananas, Beef Liver, Beets, Beet Greens, Black Cherries, Blueberries, Blue Cohosh, Birch, Broccoli, Brussels Sprouts, Cantaloupe, Carrots, Cashews, Chamomile, Citrus Fruits, Clams, Coltsfoot, Comfrey, Crab, Cucumbers, Dandelion, Dates, Dried Apricots, Dulse, Egg Whites, Eyebright, Fennel, Figs (Dried), Goat Milk, Grapes, Halibut, Irish Moss, Kelp, Mint Leaves, Milk and Dairy Products except Cheese, Mistletoe, Mullein, Nettles, Olives, Oysters, Papaya, Parsley, Peaches, Pears, Peanut Butter, Peppermint, Plantain, Pork, Potatoes, Poultry, Primrose, Raisins, Raspberry, Sage Tea, Salmon, Shepard's Purse, Spinach, Sunflower Seeds, Tomatoes, Tuna, Turnips, Veal, Vegetables, Walnuts, Watercress, Wheat Germ, White Oak Bark, Whole Grains and Cereals, Wintergreen, Yarrow | Blood, Heat, Kidneys, Muscles, Nerves, Skin |

Selenium	Beef Heart and Liver, Bran, Brazil Nuts, Brewer's Yeast, Broccoli, Brown Rice, Clams, Garlic, Kelp, Milk, Most Seaweeds, Mushrooms, Onions, Pineapples, Saltwater Fish, Soybeans, Tomatoes, Wheat Germ	Blood, Cell, Kidneys, Liver, Pancreas, Prostate Gland, Spleen, Testicles, Tissues
Silicon	Alfalfa, Almonds, Apples, Apricots, Asparagus, Bananas, Barley, Beans, Beets, Beet Greens, Blue Cohosh, Burdock, Cabbage, Cauliflower, Celery, Cherries, Chickweed, Corn, Corn Silk, Cucumbers, Dandelion Greens, Dates, Figs, Flaxseed, Grapes, Horsetail, Kelp, Kohlrabi, Millet, Nectarines, Nettles, Oats, Onions, Parsnips, Peanuts, Plums, Poppy Seed, Raisins, Raspberry, Rice (Brown or Wild), Rice (Bran or Syrup), Spinach, Sprouted Seeds, Oats (Steel-Cut), Strawberries, Sunflower Seeds, Sweet Potatoes, Tomatoes, Turnips, Wheat Bran-Germ, Whole Grains or Wheat	Bones, Hair, Nails, Teeth

Sodium	Alfalfa, Apple Tree Bark, Apples, Apricots, Asparagus, Barley, Beef, Beets and Greens, Cabbage (Red), Carrots, Celery, Cheeses, Chicken, Cleavers, Coconut, Dandelion, Dates, Dill, Dried Beef, Dulse, Eggs, Fennel, Figs, Fish, Goat Milk, Horseradish, Irish Moss, Kale, Kelp, Kidney, Milk, Mistletoe, Nettles, Okra, Olives (Black), Parsley, Pork, Prunes, Raisins, Romaine Lettuce, Saltwater Fish, Sea Salt, Sesame Seed, Shellfish, Shepard's Purse, Spinach, Strawberries, Sunflower Seeds, Thyme, Turnips, Watermelon, Whey	Blood, Lymph System, Muscles, Nerves, Stomach
Sulphur	Alfalfa, Asparagus, Avocados, Beef, Black Currant, Brazil Nuts, Broccoli, Brussels Sprouts, Burdock, Cabbage, Carrots, Cauliflower, Cayenne, Celery, Chestnuts, Coltsfoot, Corn, Cucumber, Dill, Eggs, Eyebright, Fennel, Figs, Filberts, Fish, Garlic, Horseradish, Kale, Kelp, Kohlrabi, Lima Beans, Marjoram, Milk, Mullein, Nettles, Oats, Onions, Parsley, Peas, Plantain, Poultry, Potatoes, Radish, Raspberry, Red Currants, Sage, Shepard's Purse, Soybeans, Snap Beans, Spinach, Thyme, Tomatoes, Turnip,	Hair, Nails, Nerves, Skin
Vanadium	Cucumber Peels, Fish, Lettuce, Parsley, Radishes, Strawberries	Blood Vessels, Heart

Zinc	Beef and Pork Liver, Beets and Beet Tops, Brewer's Yeast, Carrots, Cheese, Clams, Crab, Green Leafy Vegetables, Herring, Kelp, Lamb Chops, Lean Beef, Lobster, Marshmallow, Milk, Nuts, Onions, Peas, Pork Loin, Poultry, Pumpkin Seeds, Sardines, Sprouted Seeds, Sunflower Seeds, Wheat Bran and Germ	Blood, Bone, Brain, Heart, Liver, Muscle, Prostate Gland
Other Supplements	**Natural Sources**	**Affected Components**
Acidophilus	Natural "live" yogurt	Bowel, Intestines, Kidney, Sexual Organs, Skin
Antler Horn	Powered Deer or Elk Horns	Blood, Immune System, Intestines, Sexual Organs
Bee Pollen	Unpasteurized honey contains small amounts of bee pollen. Bee pollen contains protein, amino acids, sugar, and small amounts of vitamins, minerals, and enzymes	The entire body
Bioflavonoid	Apricots, Broccoli, Central White Core of Lemons, Limes, Oranges, Cherries, Citrus Fruit Peel, Green Peppers	Arteries, Capillaries, Veins
Brewer's Yeast	From hops, a by-product of beer	Lymph Nodes, Neural System, Skin

Cellulose	Apples, Bran, Brussels Sprouts, Cabbage, Carrots, Cucumber Skins, Green Beans, Peas, Peppers	Colon and Large Bowel
Charcoal	Burned cellulose, peat, wood, and bituminous coal	Blood, Intestines
Chlorophyll	Barley leaves or Algae and Chlorella	Blood, Cells, Immune System, Intestines
Co-enzyme	Beef and Beef Hearts, Beet Leaves, Peanuts, Pork, Poultry, Sardines, Spinach	All Body Cells
DHEA (Hormone)	Mexican Wild Yam	Blood, Heart, Immune System, Nervous System, Veins
Dietary Fiber	Products made from Apples, Broccoli, Brussels Sprouts, Carrots, Green Beans, Nuts, Wax Beans, and Whole Grain Cereal and Bread	Blood, Intestines
Digestive Enzymes	Avocados, Bananas, Mangoes	Blood, Cells, Organs, Tissues
Evening Primrose Oil	Seeds from Evening Primrose	Liver, Lymph Glands, Skin Cells
Glandulars	Beef and Pork	Blood, Lungs, Muscles
Lecithin	Cabbage, Cauliflower, Egg Yolks, Fish, Liver, Meat, Soybeans	Blood, Heart Liver, Nerves

Propolis	A sticky mixture containing balsam oil, pollen, resin, and wax collected by bees to fill the cracks in their hives	Blood, Immune System
Royal Jelly	Secreted by salivary glands of the worker bees to develop and nurture the queen bee	Immune System, Neural System, Sexual Organs (Male & Female, Skin
Shark Cartilage	Ground cartilage extracted from sharks	Bone, Lymph Nodes, Muscle, Sexual Organs, Skin
Seaweed	Seaweeds are a natural form of Iodine.	Glands, Intestines
Spirulina	Spirulina plankton or Blue-Green Algae	The Entire Body

Protein	Niacin	Vitamin A	Vitamin B-2	Vitamin B-6
Chicken	Salmon	Liver	Liver	Soybeans
Dry Soybeans	Tuna	Dark Green Leafy Vegetables	Organic Meats	Fresh Salmon
Fish	Chicken	Cantaloupe	Mushrooms	Ham
Ham	Halibut	Sweet Potatoes	Milk	Pork
Pork	Liver	Carrots	Whole Milk	Canned Salmon
Beef	Beef	Spinach	Brewer's Yeast	Brewer's Yeast
Vegetable Patty	Organic Meats	Chard	Fortified Cereals	Molasses
Cottage Cheese	Peanuts	Tomatoes	Eggs	Liver
	All Bran	Eggs	Beef	Wheat Bran
	Mushrooms		Cottage Cheese	Beef
	Brewer's Yeast		Chicken	Cod
	Other Fish		Spinach	Wheat Germ
			Ham	Sunflower Seeds
			Pork	

Vitamin C	Polyun-saturated Fat	Biotin	Vitamin B-1	Vitamin B-13/ Orotc Acid
Guava	Sunflower Oil	Egg yolks	Brewer's Yeast	Organically-Grown Root Vegetables
Broccoli	Corn Oil	Liver	Pork	Whey
Green Peppers	Soybean Oil	Unpolished Rice	Dry Soybeans	Curdled Milk
Brussels Sprouts	Cottonseed Oil	Brewer's Yeast	Ham	Vanadium
Cantaloupe	English Walnuts	Whole Grains	Wheat Germ	Fish
Dark Green Leafy Vegetables	Sunflower Seeds	Sardines	Sunflower Seeds	
Citrus Fruit or Juice	Margarine containing Liquid Vegetable Oil	Legumes	Fortified Cereals	
Fresh Strawberries			Brazil Nuts	
Cabbage				
Watermelon				
Vitamin D	**Vitamin E**	**Choline**	**Pantothenic Acid**	**Vitamin B-12**
Salmon	Soybean Oil	Egg Yolks	Liver	Liver Beef
Sardines	Corn or Cottonseed Oil	Organic Meats	Organic Meats	Kidney
Herring	Wheat Germ	Brewer's Yeast	Eggs	Beef
Vitamin D-Fortified Milk and Milk Products	Peanuts	Wheat Germ	Soybeans	Oysters
Egg Yolks	Margarine	Soybeans	Broccoli	Salmon
Organic Meats	Mayo	Fish	Peanuts	Fresh sole Filet
	Broiled Salmon Steak	Legumes	Mushroom	Ham
		Lecithin	Beef	Pork
			Haddock	Chicken
			Brewer's Yeast	

Folacin	Inositol	Calcium	Water	Carbohydrates
Chicken or Beef Liver	Whole Grains	Milk	Beverages	Whole Grains
Wheat Germ	Citrus Fruits	Broccoli	Fruits	Honey
Asparagus	Brewer's Yeast	Dark Green Leafy Vegetables	Vegetables	Syrup
Lettuce	Molasses	Cheese		Fruits
Spinach	Meat	Molasses		Vegetables
Orange Juice	Milk	Legumes		
Legumes	Nuts	Almonds		
	Vegetables	Cottage Cheese		
	Lecithin	Brazil Nuts		
Vitamin F	**Laetrile**	**Vitamin K**	**Pangamic Acid**	**Para-Aminobenzioic Acid**
Vegetable Oils	Whole Kernels of Apricots	Green Leafy Vegetables	Brewer's Yeast	Organic Meats
Butter	Apples	Egg Yolks	Rare Steaks	Wheat Germ
Sunflower Seeds	Cherries	Safflower Oil	Brown Rice	Yogurt
		Blackstrap Molasses	Sunflower	Molasses
		Cauliflower	Pumpkin and Sesame seeds	Green Leafy Vegetables
		Soybeans		

Vitamin P	Manganese	Selenium	Cobalt	Molybdenum
Citrus Fruits	Whole Grains	Tuna	Organic Meats	Legumes
Fruits	Green Leafy Vegetables	Herring	Oysters	Whole Grain Cereals
Black Currants	Legumes	Brewer's Yeast	Clams	Milk
Buckwheat	Nuts	Wheat Germ and Bran	Poultry	Liver
	Pineapples	Broccoli	Milk	Dark Green Vegetables
	Egg Yolks	Whole Grains	Green Leafy Vegetables	
			Fruits	

Magnesium	Potassium	Iron	Tryptophan	Phenylalanine
Soybeans	Soybeans	Prune Juice	Beef	Soy Protein
Wheat Germ	Cantaloupe	Liver	Soy Protein	Beef
Cashews	Sweet Potatoes	Beef	Chicken	Chicken
Almonds	Avocadoes	Soybeans	Soybeans	Soybeans
Brazil Nuts	Raisins	Baked Beans	Fish	Fish
Baked Beans	Bananas	Ham	Eggs	Vegetable Patty
Peanuts	Halibut	Organic Meats	Vegetable Patty	Eggs
Molasses	Sole	Chicken	Cottage Cheese	Cottage Cheese
Dark Green Leafy Vegetables	Baked Beans	Spinach	Milk	Baked Beans
	Molasses	Eggs	Mixed Nuts	Peanuts
	Ham		Baked Beans	Almonds
	Mushrooms			Milk
	Beef			
	White Potatoes			

Leucine	Sodium	Copper	Zinc	Phosphorus
Beef	Seafood	Organic Meats	Beef	Tuna
Chicken	Table Salt	Seafood	Oatmeal	Sweetbreads
Soy Protein	Baking Powder	Nuts	Dark Chicken	Wheat Germ
Fish	Baking Soda	Legumes	Fish	Soybeans
Soybeans	Celery	Molasses	Beef Liver	Fried Beef Liver
Ham	Processed Foods	Raisins	Dried Beans	Brazil Nuts
Pork	Milk Products	Bone Meal	Bran	Beef
Cottage Cheese	Kelp		Tuna	Skim Milk
Liver				Processed Cheese
Vegetable Patty				
Eggs				
Baked Beans				

Sulphur	Iodine	Vitamin T	Vitamin U	Chromium
Fish	Iodized Salt	Sesame Seeds	Raw Cabbage Juice	Corn Oil
Eggs	Ocean Fish	Raw Sesame Butter	Fresh Cabbage	Clams
Meats	Shellfish	Egg Yolks	Home-made Sauerkraut	Whole Grain Cereals
Cabbage	Spinach			Brewer's Yeast
Brussels Sprouts				

Chlorine	Fluoride	Vanadium	Iso-Leucine	Lysine
Table Salt	Tea	Fish	Beef	Chicken
Seafood	Seafood		Chicken	Beef
Meats	Bone Meal		Fish	Fish
Ripe Olives			Soybeans	Ham
Rye Flour			Soy Protein	Pork
			Ham	Soy Protein
			Pork	Soybeans
			Vegetable Patty	Cottage Cheese
			Eggs	Baked Beans
			Cottage Cheese	Eggs
			Liver	Goat Milk
			Baked Beans	Milk
			Milk	Peanuts
				Vegetable Patty
				Brewer's Yeast

Valine	Methionine	Threonine		
Beef	Chicken	Beef		
Chicken	Beef	Chicken,		
Fish	Fish	Fish,		
Soy Protein	Soy Protein	Ham		
Soybeans	Soybeans	Pork		
Ham	Ham	Soy Protein		
Pork	Pork	Soybeans		
Eggs	Eggs	Liver		
Liver	Liver	Eggs		
Vegetable Patty	Vegetable Patty	Cottage Cheese		
Cottage Cheese	Cottage Cheese	Goat Milk		
Baked Beans	Baked Beans	Baked Beans		
Milk	Milk	Vegetable Patty		

Foods High In Refined Sugar		Food High in Sugar	
Ready-to-Serve Breakfast Cereals	Ice Milk	Sweetened and Sugar- Coated Cereals	Instant Breakfast
White Bread	Sherbet	Cakes and Icings	Breakfast Squares
Pancakes	Fruit, Canned or Frozen in Syrup	Cookies	Sweet Pickles
Cakes and Icings	Sweetened Applesauce	Pies	
Cookies and Pies	Syrups and Sweet Sauces	Bran Muffins	Sweetened Yogurt
Rolls and Muffins	Jams and Jellies	Graham Crackers	Jello
Sandwich Buns and English Muffins	Candy and Chocolate	Sweet Rolls	Puddings
		Coffee Cakes	Custards
Biscuits	Jello	Doughnuts	Hot Chocolate
Saltines and Graham Crackers	Puddings and Custards	Ice Cream	Chocolate Milk
	Sweetened Yogurt	Ice Milk	
Pretzels	Instant Breakfast	Sherbet	Milkshakes
Macaroni Noodles and Spaghetti	Breakfast Squares	Fruit, Canned or Frozen in Syrup	Ovaltine
	Hot Chocolate	Sweetened Applesauce	Kool-Aid
Sweet Rolls	Milkshakes		Tang
Doughnuts and Pop Tarts	Ovaltine	Sweet Potatoes Candied or in Syrup	Canned or Frozen Fruit Drinks
Coffee Cakes	Soft Drinks		
White and Instant Rice	Kool-Aid	Chocolate Sauce	Soft Drinks
	Tang and Fruit drinks	Other Sweet Sauces and Syrups	Popsicles
Flour Tortillas			Dessert Wines and Cordials
Cream Sauces and Soups	Popsicles	Jams and Jellies	
	Beer and Wine	Candy including: Candy Bars	
Candied Sweet Potatoes	Hard Liquor		
	Brandy and Cordials	Hard candy	
Sweet Pickles		Life Savers	
Snack Foods		Cough Drops	
Ice Cream		Chocolate	

List of Plaque-Forming Foods			
Sweetened and Sugar-Coated Cereals	Coffee Cakes	Instant Breakfast	Candy
Oatmeal	Doughnuts	Breakfast Squares	Chocolate
Pancakes	Ice Cream	Hot Chocolate	Thousand Island Dressing
Cakes and Icings	Ice Milk	Milkshakes	Sweetened Yogurt
Cookies	Sherbet	Ovaltine	Jello
Pies	Fruit, Canned or Frozen Syrup	Jams and Jellies	Puddings
Graham Crackers	Fruit, Canned (Sugar-Free)	Syrups and Sweet Sauces	Custards
Sweet Rolls			

SHOPPING GUIDE

HEALTHY SHOPPING TIPS: Add vegetables, spices, and herbs to your meals.

Turmeric and basil help prevent cancer of the bladder and prostate.

Jalapenos, hot peppers, black pepper, and mustard boost your metabolism and burn fat.

Cinnamon (great in teas) helps metabolize sugar, and keeps blood sugar levels regulated.

Onion and garlic boost the immune system.

Parsley oxygenates the blood system.

Azure Standard
Organic Herb Farms, Dried Herb Suppliers, and Formula Sources
Phone: (541) 467-2230
Website: www.azurestandard.com

Herb n' Essences
Organically-Grown and Wild-Harvested Herbal Preparations
Bonne Labuda
Master Herbalist
19999 Beaver Lake Road
Kimball, MN 55353-9712
Phone: (320) 252-5745
Fax: (320) 253-7408
Website: www.herbnessences.com

Blessed Herbs
109 Barre Plains Road
Oakham, Massachusetts 01069
Phone: (800) 489-4372
Fax: (508) 882-3755
Email: info@blessedherbs.com
Website: www.blessedherbs.com

Mountain Rose Herbs
PO Box 50220
Eugene, Oregon 97405
Phone: (800) 879-3337
Fax: (510) 217-4012
Website: www.mountainherbs.com

Present Moments
3546 Grand Avenue South
Minneapolis, MN 55408
Phone: (800) 378-3245
Website: www.presentmoments.com

Milk
Organic Pastures (CA) -- raw whole cow's milk ... (877) RAW-MILK

Cheese
Grazin' Acres -- raw full cottage cheese ... (608) 727-2904
Green Acres Farm -- raw cottage cheese ... (717) 661-5293
Pleasant Pastures -- raw cottage cheese and cream cheese ... (717) 768-3437

Aged Cheese
Copper Creek Farm -- cow and goat cheeses ... (765) 395-7886
Farm Fromage -- cow and goat cheeses ... (717) 314-137
Meadow Ridge Farm -- goat cheese ... (717) 656-2261

Cream
Grazin' Acres -- raw cream and crème fraiche (608) 727-2904)
Rainbow Acres -- raw cream (717-442-0132)
Sustainable Living Acres -- raw cream and sour cream (717) 665-0280

Yogurt and Kefir
Green Acres ... (717) 661-5293
Grazin' Acres -- yogurt and kefir ... (608) 727-2904
Sustainable Living Acres -- buttermilk, kefir, and yogurt ... (717) 665-0280

Eggs
Copper Creek Farm ... (765) 394-7886
Meadow Ridge ... (717) 530-5999

Grazin' Acres -- soy-free fertilized pastured eggs ... (608) 727-2904
Sunny Crest Pastures -- pasteurized eggs ... (717) 768-0101

Butter

Barnville Creamery -- raw cultured butter ... (717) 656-4422
Meadow Ridge Farm -- raw goat butter ... (717) 530-5999
Honeysuckle Acres -- raw butter ... (717) 423-6429
Sunny Crest Pastures -- raw butter ... (717) 768-0101

Ice Cream

Copper Creek Farm ... (765) 395-7886
Grazin' Acres ... (608) 727-2904

Seafood

Fishhugger Wild Seafood ... (602) 286-9233
Live Superfoods -- salmon roe, wild salmon jerky ... (800) 481-5074
Vital Choice -- fresh wild salmon ... (800) 608-4825

HEALTHY TIP #18: Buy house plants (Spider plants are best)-- They oxygenate your home.

Flowering house plants boost your morale.

Fats and Oils

Green Hills Harvest -- lard ... (660) 244-5858
Prather Ranch -- pastured pork, lard ... (415) 378-2917
Tiburtini -- olive oil from Zingerman's ... (888) 636-8162
Coconut Oil Online ... (800) 922-1744

Fresh Meat

5 Bar -- beef ... (714) 749-5717
Fox Fire Farms -- lamb ... (970) 563-4675
Great Beef ... greatbeef.com
Willow Hills -- pastured poultry ... willowhills.org
Rocky Mountain Organic Meats – beef, primals, lamb, cold cuts, jerky ... www.rockymtncuts.com

Processed Meats

Caw Caw Creek -- ham, sausage, bacon ... (803) 917-0794
Green Pastures Dairy -- summer sausage ... (218) 384-4513

Uncured Natural Meats -- sausage, beef, bacon ... (920) 386-4971
Your Family Cow -- beef sausages, kielbasa ... (717) 729-9730

Pemmican and Jerky
Live Superfoods -- wild salmon, jerky ... (800) 841-5074
Northstar -- bison jerky, snack sticks ... (888) 295-6332
West Wind Farms -- beef jerky ... (423) 442-9768
Your Family Cow -- beef jerky and sticks ... (717) 729-9730

Fruits and Vegetables
Beck Grove -- biodynamic fruit ... (760) 723-9997
Frutos -- dried fruit ... (888) 565-6633
Raw from the Farm -- organic sun-dried fruit ... rawfromthefarm.
com
Walton Orchids -- biodynamic fruit ... (616) 352-7679

Lacto-Fermented Vegetables
Happy Girl Kitchen Company -- pickles ... (831) 750-9579
Immunutrition -- cultured vegetables ... (877) 773-9229
Rejuvenate Foods -- cultured vegetables ... (800) 805-7957
Zukay Live Foods -- lacto-fermented salsa ... Zukaylive.com

Lacto-Fermentation Starters
Danlac Dairy -- cultures ... (403) 948-4644
Happy Herbalist ... (888) 425-8827
Live Superfoods -- kefir and culture starters ... (800) 481-5074
The CheeseMaker -- cheese cultures ... (414) 745-5483

Grain and Legumes
Field of Grains Flours & Grains ... www.fieldofgrains.com, (763)
684-8115
Blue Mountain ... (540) 745-5040
Country Creations ... (866) 546-9297
Homegrown Harvest ... (866) 394-5954
Natural Lifestyle -- grains ... (800) 752-2775

Bread and Crackers
Grindstone Bakery ... (707) 515-6666
Miller Bakery ... (530) 532-6384

Mary's Gone Crackers ... (925) 258-1200
Glaser Sprouted Crackers ... (305) 238-7747

HEALTHY TIP #19: Posture – Good posture increases circulation to the central nervous system

Coconut Products
Desiccated coconut (in most health food stores)
Tropical Traditions -- creamed coconut ... (866) 311-2626
Glaser Organics -- fresh organic coconut water ... (305) 238-7747
Coconut sugar (also sold as palm sugar in Asian markets)

Nuts and Nut Products
Blue Mountain Organics -- nuts and nut butters ...
bluemountainorganics.com
Higher Power -- raw, sprouted nuts ... higherpower.biz
Natural Health Advocates -- soaked nut butters ... (717) 733-2634
Shiloh Farms -- raw nuts ... (800) 362-6832

Condiments
Emperor's Kitchen ... (800) 334-5809
Natural Lifestyle ... (800) 752-2775
Miller Organic ... (717) 556-0672

Salts and Spices
Celtic Sea Salt ... (800) 867-7258
Nature's Cargo Sea Salt ... (888) 725-8386
Copper Creek Farm -- seasonings ... (765) 395-7886

Soups and Stocks
Bone Werks Culinarte -- stocks ... (800) 542-3032
Green Acres Farm -- beef and chicken stock ... (717) 661-5293
Perfect Addition -- frozen stocks ... (310) 559-4770
US Wellness Meats -- beef stock ... (877) 383-0051
Rocky Mountain Organic Meats -- soup bones ...
www.rockymtncuts.com

Snack Foods
Freeland Foods GO Raw -- spirulina super chips ... (650) 962-9299
Meant To be Foods -- coconut cruffles ... (206) 604-1460
Gopal's Japanese Mexican Italian ... (866) 646-7257
High Power trail mixes ... (877) 684-8763

Cookies and Bars
Alive and Radiant Foods -- cookies and lemon swirls ... (510) 527-8916
Beccaroons -- macaroons ... (952) 451-0343
Lydia's Organics -- raspberry, spirulina, and tropical mango bars ... (415) 258-9678
Pamela's shortbread cookies

Sweeteners
Jorgan Eiden -- raw honey ... (320) 749-2481
Mascava -- organic sugar ... (800) 656-3668
Back Creek -- maple syrup ... (540) 499-2302

Beverages
Caveman Foods ... (612) 240-4810
Copper Creek Farm -- kombucha ... (765) 395-7886

Supplements
Green Pasture X-Factor -- butter oil ... (402) 338-5551
Carlson Labs -- desiccated liver ... (888) 234-5656
Immune Tree -- dried colostrum ... (888) 484-8671
Prime Directive -- probiotic ... (877) 399-3351

HEALTHY TIP #20: Bowel Movements – It's important to have at least 2 to 3 movements per day.

Add more raw fruits and vegetables to your daily diet.